Antimicrobial stewardship

Antimicrobial stewardship

Edited by

Matthew Laundy

Mark Gilchrist

Laura Whitney

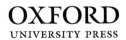

OXFORD

UNIVERSITY PRESS

OXFORD

UNIVERSITY PRESS

Great Clarendon Street, Oxford, OX2 6DP,
United Kingdom

Oxford University Press is a department of the University of Oxford.
It furthers the University's objective of excellence in research, scholarship,
and education by publishing worldwide. Oxford is a registered trade mark of
Oxford University Press in the UK and in certain other countries

First Edition published in 2016

Impression: 1

Published in the United States of America by Oxford University Press
198 Madison Avenue, New York, NY 10016, United States of America

British Library Cataloguing in Publication Data

Data available

Library of Congress Control Number: 2016934615

ISBN 978-0-19-875879-2

Printed and bound by
CPI Group (UK) Ltd, Croydon, CR0 4YY

To our children: Amelia, Freya, Jacob, and Sophie.
May our actions now make a safer future for you.

The fault, dear Brutus, is not in our stars.
But in ourselves, that we are underlings.

Julius Caesar (Act I, Sc. II)

William Shakespeare

Preface

The twentieth century has been described as the golden age of antimicrobials. With the introduction of antimicrobials previously deadly infectious diseases were relegated to history. Now in the second decade of the twenty-first century it has become increasingly obvious to even the most disinterested member of the public, healthcare professional, or politician that there is a problem with antimicrobial-resistant organisms and untreatable infections. This problem of antimicrobial resistance has been raised as a worldwide concern alongside global warming, and the popular press regularly raises the spectre of a 'return to the dark ages'.

While resistance is an inevitable evolutionary process, two factors have accelerated the development of untreatable infections. Firstly the pharmaceutical industry had lost interest in antimicrobial development, primarily for financial reasons, and so there are fewer new classes of antimicrobials in the pipeline as a consequence. The second is the overuse and abuse of antimicrobials by the medical profession, the public, and the agricultural industry.

The concept of antimicrobial stewardship has been developing within the infection community over the last 15 years. The aim of antimicrobial stewardship is to restrict antimicrobial use in order to reduce the development of resistance, avoid the side effects associated with antimicrobial use, and optimize clinical outcomes. In its simplest form it's about saving what antimicrobials we have.

This is a rapidly developing field. The number of academic papers on antimicrobial stewardship has increased dramatically in the past 5 years, from 43 in 2008 to 429 in 2015.

Our aim is to produce a very practical approach to antimicrobial stewardship. It's very much a 'how to' guide supported by a review of the available evidence.

The book is divided into three sections.

Section 1: Setting the scene and starting up: in this section we look at the problem of antimicrobial resistance, problems in the antimicrobial supply line, and initiatives to improve the situation. We examine the psychological, social, cultural, and organizational factors in antimicrobial use and prescribing. We look at the principles and goals of antimicrobial stewardship. Finally we look at how to establish an antimicrobial stewardship programme.

Section 2: Components of an antimicrobial stewardship programme: in this section we examine the identified components of an antimicrobial stewardship programme—prospective audit and feedback, antimicrobial policies and formularies, antimicrobial restriction, intravenous to oral switch, measuring antimicrobial consumption, and measuring and feeding back stewardship; we conclude with a look at information technology in antimicrobial stewardship.

Section 3: Special areas in antimicrobial stewardship: in this section we explore specific areas of antimicrobial stewardship including antimicrobial pharmacokinetics and dynamics, intensive care units, paediatrics, surgical prophylaxis, near-patient testing, and infection biomarkers. We will also look at antimicrobial stewardship in the community and long-term care facilities, where arguably there is most to be done. We conclude the book by looking at antimicrobial stewardship in resource-poor settings and the unique challenges facing low- and middle-income countries.

Infection control is a vital component in the control of the spread of resistant organisms. We will touch on aspects of infection control, but there are many textbooks that can cover this subject in far more detail that we are able to here. We will not cover the exact mechanisms of antimicrobial resistance as this field is rapidly developing and the book would soon be out of date, nor is this a pharmacology book on antimicrobials. The issue of the widespread use of antimicrobials in the livestock industry, while critical to the control of resistance, is beyond the control of the intended audience of this book and will not be covered.

The primary audience for this book comprises infection trainees and specialists from the medical, pharmacy, nursing, and scientific professions. It will also be of interest to those in the professions outside infection. Policy makers and commissioners of services will find this book useful to help inform policy and ensure the commissioning of high-quality services. Antimicrobials and infection training are paradoxically forming an ever smaller part of the undergraduate medical curriculum and medical students may find this book useful for filling in their knowledge gaps. Ultimately, antimicrobial resistance is everyone's problem and we hope this book will appeal to a broad audience.

Contents

Abbreviations and glossary

A&F	audit and feedback	C_{max}	maximum antibiotic concentration
ABW	adjusted body weight	C_p	antibiotic concentration in plasma
ABX	antibiotic		
ADQ	average daily quantity	CPE	carbapenemase-producing *Enterobacteriaceae*
ADR	adverse drug reaction		
AFS	antifungal stewardship	CRE	carbapenem-resistant *Enterobacteriaceae*
AMR	antimicrobial resistance		
AMS	antimicrobial stewardship	CRO	carbapenem-resistant organism
AMT	antimicrobial management team	CRP	C-reactive protein
		CVC	central venous catheter
ARPEC	Antibiotic Resistance and Prescribing in European Children	DDD	defined daily dose
		DID	defined daily dose per 1000 inhabitants per day
ASP	antimicrobial stewardship programme	DOT	days of therapy
AST	antimicrobial susceptibility test(ing)/antimicrobial stewardship team	EARS-Net	European Antimicrobial Resistance Surveillance Network
ASTRO-PU	age, sex, and temporary resident originated prescribing unit	ECDC	European Centre for Disease Prevention and Control
		EHR	electronic health record
ATC	Anatomical Therapeutic Chemical Classification System	EMR	electronic medical record
		EPR	electronic patient record
AUC	area under the concentration–time curve	ESAC	European Surveillance of Antimicrobial Consumption
BMI	body mass index	ESBL	extended spectrum β-lactamase
BRICS	Brazil, Russia, India, China, and South Africa	ESPAUR	English Surveillance Programme on Antimicrobial Usage and Resistance
BSAC	British Society for Antimicrobial Chemotherapy	ESVAC	European Surveillance of Veterinary Antibiotic Consumption
C&BI	clinical and business intelligence		
		ETGA	enzymatic template generation and amplification
CAP	community-acquired pneumonia	EU	European Union
CCG	Clinical Commissioning Group, a local NHS(UK) commissioning body	EUCAST	European Committee on Antimicrobial Susceptibility Testing
CDC	Centers for Disease Control (Atlanta, GA, USA)	GARP	Global Antibiotic Resistance Partnership
CDI	*Clostridium difficile* infection	GDP	gross domestic product
CDSS	clinical decision support system	GHSA	Global Health Security Agenda
CL	clearance	GI	gastrointestinal

GP	general practitioner
HAART	highly active antiretroviral therapy
HAP	hospital-acquired pneumonia
HCAI	healthcare-associated infection
HCW	healthcare worker
HEPA	high-efficiency particulate air (filter)
Hib	*Haemophilus influenzae* serotype b
HIMSS	Healthcare Information and Management Systems Society
HIV	human immunodeficiency virus
HL7	Health Level 7—a standard framework for exchange of electronic health information
HSCT	haematopoietic stem-cell transplantation
iCCM	integrated community case management
ICU	intensive care unit
ID	infectious disease
IDSA	Infectious Disease Society of America
IFI	invasive fungal infection
IHI	Institute for Healthcare Improvement
IMAI	integrated management of adolescent and adult illness
IMCI	integrated management of childhood illness
INF	infection
IP&C	infection prevention and control
ITU	intensive therapy unit
IV	intravenous
IVOST	intravenous to oral antibiotic switch therapy
LBW	lean body weight
LMICs	low- and middle-income countries
LMS	laboratory management system
LOS	length of stay
LTCF	long-term care facilities
MALDI-TOF-MS	matrix-assisted laser desorption ionization time-of-flight mass spectrometry

MASCC	Multinational Association for Supportive Care in Cancer
MDRO	multidrug-resistant organisms
MDT	multidisciplinary team
Medical infection specialist	a medically qualified specialist in microbiology or infectious disease. A term used to reflect differing roles of medical microbiologists across the world, in some countries being primarily laboratory based while in other countries having more ward and patient-facing roles
MIC	minimum inhibitory concentration
MODS	multiple organ dysfunction syndrome
MOOC	massive open online course
MRSA	meticillin-resistant *Staphylococcus aureus*
NHS	National Health Service (UK)
NICE	National Institute for Health and Care Excellence (a body that provides national guidance and advice to improve health and social care in England and Wales)
NICU	neonatal intensive care
NNT	number needed to treat
NPfIT	National Program for IT (a UK programme for roll-out of IT across the NHS)
OPAT	outpatient parenteral antibiotic therapy
OTC	over-the-counter
PASP	paediatric antimicrobial stewardship programme
PBR	payment by results
PCR	polymerase chain reaction
PCT	procalcitonin
PCT	Primary Care Trust (a local healthcare commissioning and provider body within the UK NHS, now defunct. Commissioning role now replaced by CCGs)
PD	pharmacodynamics
PHE	Public Health England

PICU	paediatric intensive care unit
PIL	patient information leaflet
PK	pharmacokinetics
PNA FISH	peptide nucleic acid fluorescent *in situ* hybridization
POC(T)	point of care (testing)
PPS	point prevalence survey
PRISMS	Prescribing Information System for Scotland
QIP	quality improvement programme
QIPP	quality, innovation, productivity, and prevention
QOF	quality outcome frameworks
RTI	respiratory tract infection
SAASP	South African Antibiotic Stewardship Programme
SAPG	The Scottish Antimicrobial Prescribing Group
SCIP	Surgical Care Improvement Project
ScotMARAP 2	Scottish Management of AMR Action Plan 2
ScRAP	Scottish Reduction in AMR
SIGN	Scottish Intercollegiate Guideline Network
SOT	solid organ transplantation
SSI	surgical site infection

STAR	Strategy for Tackling Antimicrobial Resistance
STAR	Stemming the Tide of Antibiotic Resistance
STAR-PU	specific therapeutic group age–sex weightings related prescribing units
TARGET	Treat Antibiotics Responsibly, Guidelines, Education, Tools
TATFAR	Transatlantic Taskforce on Antimicrobial Resistance
TB	tuberculosis
TBW	total body weight
TDM	therapeutic drug monitoring
UCS	urgent care services
UK	United Kingdom
UK-VARSS	UK Veterinary Antibiotic Resistance and Sales Surveillance
USA	United States
USD	United States dollar
UTI	urinary tract infection
Vd	volume of distribution
VRE	vancomycin-resistant *Enterococcus*
WARP-SU	Welsh Antimicrobial Resistance Programme Surveillance Unit
WHA	World Health Assembly
WHO	World Health Organization

Contributors

Dr Jonathan Ball MRCP EDIC FCCP
FFICM MSc MD
Consultant and Honorary Senior Lecturer in
General and Neuro Intensive Care, St George's
University Hospitals NHS Foundation Trust,
London, UK

Dr Julia Bielicki MB/BChir MD MPH
Clinical Research Fellow, Paediatric
Infectious Diseases Research Group, Institute
for Infection and Immunity, St George's,
University of London, London, UK

Dr Tihana Bicanic BM BCh
MD(Res) MRCP
Consultant in Infectious Diseases, St George's
University Hospitals NHS Foundation Trust;
Reader in Infectious Diseases, Institute
for Infection and Immunity, St George's,
University of London, London, UK

Dr Gabriel Birgand PharmD MPH PhD
Research Associate, NIHR Health Protection
Research Unit, Healthcare Associated
Infection and Antimicrobial Resistance,
Imperial College London, Hammersmith
Campus, UK

Esmita Charani MPharm MSc Diploma in
Infectious Diseases
Academic Research Pharmacist, NIHR
Health Protection Research Unit, Healthcare
Associated Infection and Antimicrobial
Resistance, Imperial College London,
Hammersmith Campus, UK

Dr Menino Osbert Cotta BPharm
(Hons) PhD
Associate Lecturer, School of Pharmacy and
Burns Trauma and Critical Care Research
Centre, The University of Queensland; Senior
Pharmacist, Royal Brisbane and Women's
Hospital, Brisbane, Australia

Patrick Doyle BSc(Hons) (Pharmacy and
Pharmacology) MRPharmS
Pharmacy CG and Risk Lead, Frimley Health
NHS Foundation Trust, Wexham Park, UK

Dr Matthew Dryden MD FRCPath
Consultant Microbiologist and Infection
Specialist, Hampshire Hospitals Foundation
Trust, Winchester, UK; Rare and Imported
Pathogens Laboratory, Public Health
England, Porton Down, Salisbury, UK;
Southampton University School of Medicine,
Southampton, UK

Dr Naomi Fleming BPharm MRPharmS
PGDip PhD
Kettering General Hospital, Kettering, UK;
UKCPA PIN Committee

Mark Gilchrist MPharm MSc IPres FFRPS
Consultant Pharmacist Infectious Diseases,
Imperial College Healthcare NHS Trust;
Honorary Lecturer, Imperial College
London, UK

Dr Susan Hopkins
Consultant in Infectious Diseases and
Microbiology, Royal Free London NHS
Foundation Trust, UK; Healthcare
Epidemiologist, Public Health England, UK;
Honorary Senior Lecturer, University College
London, London, UK

Mr Simon Jameson PhD FRCS (Tr&Orth)
Robin Ling Hip Fellow; Princess Elizabeth
Orthopaedic Centre; Royal Devon and Exeter
NHS Foundation Trust, Exeter, UK

Dr Matthew Laundy BPharm
MBBCh MSc FRCPath MRCPCH
Consultant in Medical Microbiology,
Clinical Lead for Antimicrobial Stewardship;
St George's University Hospitals NHS
Foundation Trust, London, UK; Honorary
Senior Lecturer, Institute for Infection and
Immunity; St George's, University of London,
London, UK

Haifa Lyster MSc FFRPS MRPharmS
Consultant Pharmacist—Transplantation
and VADs, Royal Brompton and Harefield
NHS Foundation Trust, London, UK

William Malcolm BSc MSc MPH
Pharmaceutical Adviser, NHS National
Services Scotland, UK

Professor Marc Mendelson BSc PhD MBBS
FRCP(UK) DTM&H
Professor of Infectious Diseases, Head
of Division of Infectious Diseases and
HIV Medicine, Department of Medicine,
University of Cape Town, Groote Schuur
Hospital, Cape Town, South Africa

Dr Tamsin Oswald MBChB MRCP FRCPath
Northumbria Healthcare NHS Foundation
Trust, UK

Dr Sanjay Patel MA, MSc, MBBS, MRCPCH
Consultant in Paediatric Infectious Diseases
and Immunology, Southampton Children's
Hospital, Southampton, UK

Mr Mike Reed MD FRCS(T&O)
Institute of Cellular Medicine, University of
Newcastle and Northumbria Healthcare NHS
Foundation Trust, UK

Dr Peter Riley MD FRCPath
Consultant Medical Microbiologist,
St George's University Hospitals NHS
Foundation Trust; Honorary Senior Lecturer,
St George's, University of London, London, UK

Professor Jason Roberts PhD BPharm (Hons)
BAppSc FSHP
NHMRC Career Development Fellow, Burns
Trauma and Critical Care Research Centre,
The University of Queensland; Pharmacist
Consultant, Royal Brisbane and Women's
Hospital, Brisbane, Australia

Ms Fiona Robb MPharm MSc MRPharmS
Antimicrobial Pharmacist, NHS Greater
Glasgow and Clyde Health Board, Queen
Elizabeth University Hospital, Glasgow, UK

Dr Antonia Scobie MBBS BSc MSc MRCP
FRPCPath DTM&H
Specialist Registrar in Microbiology and
Infectious Diseases, St George's University
Hospitals NHS Foundation Trust, London, UK

Dr Andrew Seaton MBChB DTM&H MD
FRCP (Edinburgh and Glasgow)
Consultant in Infectious Diseases and General
Medicine and Antimicrobial Management
Team lead NHS Greater Glasgow and
Clyde Health Board, UK; Queen Elizabeth
University Hospital, Glasgow, UK

Dr Jacqueline Sneddon MRPharmS MSc
PhD, FFRPS
Project Lead for Scottish Antimicrobial
Prescribing Group, Healthcare Improvement
Scotland, UK

Dr Hayley Wickens BPharm(Hons) MSc PhD
FFRPS
Consultant Pharmacist, Anti-infectives,
University Hospital Southampton NHS
Foundation Trust, Southampton, UK

Laura Whitney MPharm MSc MRPS
Consultant Pharmacist, Antimicrobials
and Pharmacy Lead for Antimicrobial
Stewardship, St George's University Hospitals
NHS Foundation Trust; Honorary Senior
Lecturer, Kingston University, London, UK

Section 1

Setting the scene and starting up

Chapter 1

The international and national challenges faced in ensuring prudent use of antibiotics

Susan Hopkins

Introduction to the challenges faced in ensuring prudent use of antibiotics

Antimicrobial resistance (AMR) is a natural phenomenon in which microbes evolve and develop traits that enable them to survive exposure to antimicrobial agents. In the past, the problem of resistance to antimicrobials was addressed by developing new agents to which clinically important pathogens were not (at least initially) resistant. There is a relative lack of new antimicrobials that are likely to become available for use in the near future; for example, there are only three antibiotics in development at present that could potentially be active against multidrug-resistant Gram-negative bacteria. Therefore the priority is to understand the challenges of AMR and consider methods whereby healthcare organizations, public health researchers, policy makers, and the public can prudently use the antimicrobials that are currently available to prevent the apocalyptic scenario of pan-resistance.

Despite the decline in mortality rates from infectious diseases, the burden of disease and the economic impact of infections and infectious diseases, estimated to be approximately £30 billion each year in England, remain high. The presence of AMR challenges the treatment of clinical infections. These infections are more difficult to eliminate or contain in the host, resulting in poorer treatment outcomes, longer hospital inpatient stays, and increased mortality [1]. Recent English data showed that *Escherichia coli* bloodstream infections that were resistant to ciprofloxacin were associated with increased mortality [2]. Additionally, modern medicine, which includes complex surgical procedures and cancer treatments, is reliant on effective antibiotics to treat and prevent infections. Antibiotics are unusual in that the inappropriate use of antibiotics has a negative effect not only on the individual taking the medication but also, through ecological pressure, throughout society, with impacts on the emergence and spread of bacteria.

In 2013, more than 50% of children worldwide who died before the age of 5 died from infectious causes [3]. The burden of AMR and its societal cost are expected to continue to rise unless significant progress is made in preventing infections and developing diagnostics and new drugs to treat infections. A recent economic analysis estimated that unless we take the right steps to control AMR soon, a continued rise in resistance by 2050 may lead to 10 million people dying prematurely every year, with an estimated 300 million deaths by 2050 unless the current trajectory is halted. The report also estimated a 2–3.5% reduction in the world's gross domestic product (GDP) in 2050, with a cost of approximately USD 100 trillion [4].

In the UK, the scale of the threat of AMR and the case for action were set out in the 'Annual report of the Chief Medical Officer 2011', published in March 2013 [5]. In response, the government published the 'UK five year antimicrobial resistance strategy 2013 to 2018' in September 2013 [6]. This cross-government strategy sets out seven key areas of action to address AMR. The World Health Organization (WHO) is in the process of developing a global action plan on AMR, which was endorsed by the World Health Assembly (WHA) in May 2015. The Global Health Security Agenda (GHSA), launched in 2014 by the US government, has recognized antimicrobial resistance as one of four key risks to global health [7].

The focus of this chapter is antibacterial resistance and stewardship, as this is recognized as the largest current threat. The same principles of resistance and stewardship, however, can be applied to antifungals, antivirals, and antiprotozoals.

How do bacteria become resistant?

AMR is the ability of microorganisms to grow in the presence of a drug that was previously able to kill them or limit their growth. Some bacteria are naturally resistant to certain antibiotics as they lack the drug's target structure. This is called intrinsic or innate resistance. Acquired or extrinsic resistance results from the acquisition of mutations, usually occurring during multiplication (more common in viruses with single point mutations conferring resistance) or through the spread of genes on mobile genetic elements such as plasmids. The multiplication and transmission of resistance genes in and between bacterial species can occur directly through conjugation or during cell lysis or transduction when bacterial cells are infected by bacteriophages.

The main mechanisms of AMR are as follows:

- enzymatic destruction, e.g. TEM beta-lactamases, extended spectrum beta-lactamases and more recently described carbapenemases in Gram-negative bacteria;
- alterations of the cell wall to prevent entry or attachment of the antimicrobial, e.g. the alteration of penicillin-binding protein 2A confers methicillin resistance in *Staphylococcus aureus*;
- increased efflux of antimicrobials if entry occurs, e.g. the MexXY multidrug efflux system in *Pseudomonas*;
- chemical modification of the antimicrobials, e.g. enzymatic modification of aminoglycosides to inactivate the molecules;
- modification of the site or the metabolic pathway targeted by the antimicrobial, e.g. bypass of the folic acid pathway in bacteria to prevent sulfa or trimethoprim antibiotics from working.

What influences the spread of resistance?

In both humans and animals, antibiotics provide selection pressure to favour the emergence of resistant strains. Resistant bacteria can spread between humans through person-to-person contact in the community, care homes, and in hospitals. Environmental reservoirs are an important vector in hospitals. Increasingly, the impacts of travel and health tourism are also recognized as a route for acquisition of resistant bacteria in humans [8]. Resistant bacteria from animals and humans can be transmitted in both directions, through human contact with live farm, wildlife, or companion animals or their environments, through preparation and ingestion of contaminated food (both imported and locally produced animal and vegetable or fruit items), and through contact with effluent waste from humans, animals, and industry through occupational and recreational activities—this is especially important where sewage is uncontrolled (Figure 1.1).

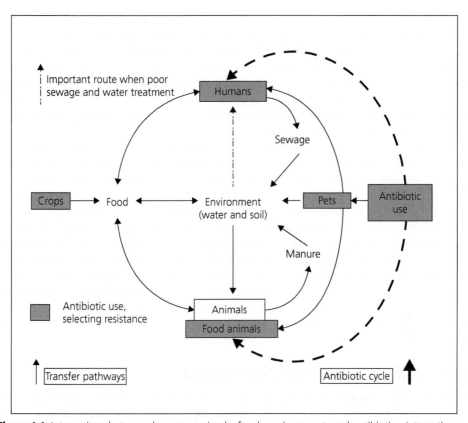

Figure 1.1 Interactions between humans, animals, food, environment, and antibiotics. Interactions occur across local, regional, national, and international boundaries with movement of humans, animals, and food within and between countries [9].

Reproduced from *ESBLs—A threat to human and animal health,* Report by the Joint Working Group of DARC and ARHAI, © Crown Copyright 2012, under the Open Government Licence v.3.0, available from https://www.gov.uk/government/uploads/system/uploads/attachment_data/file/215180/dh_132534.pdf

Many studies have demonstrated both an individual and an ecological effect between antimicrobial treatment and resistance in humans and animals. This is particularly important in care settings and among the elderly, where there is increased consumption of antibiotics. In the acute hospital setting, one in three patients is on antibiotics [10] at any point in time, with 30–50% assessed as receiving the incorrect antibiotic or not clinically requiring an antibiotic when reviewed by experts [11,12]. Eighty per cent of all antibiotics are prescribed in general practice. In the community, one in three individuals receives at least one prescription each year, rising to more than one in two in those aged over 85 years [13]. In community care homes, one in twenty individuals is on an antibiotic at any time. In the developing world, uncontrolled antibiotic sales and inadequate doses and durations of therapy all produce the perfect storm for the selection of resistance.

The importance of surveillance

Surveillance of AMR is required to track emerging drug resistance, monitor the susceptibility of microorganisms to antimicrobials, and define AMR phenotypes (expression) and genotypes (molecular DNA). It is necessary to inform the scale of the problem, assess trends, evaluate the public health burden of AMR in the population, and monitor the impact of interventions aimed to minimize the spread and burden of AMR. Dissemination of information from AMR surveillance improves infection treatment guidelines on the correct antibiotics to use in patients to prevent complications. A recent WHO report highlighted the lack of robust global AMR surveillance: of the 194 member states, 114 (58.7%) returned data on at least one of the nine areas and only 22 (11%) were able to provide data on all nine combinations requested, with the largest gaps being in Africa, the Middle East, and European states outside the European Union.

Antibiotic sales worldwide are of the order of USD 40 billion annually. The gathering of antimicrobial consumption data allows comparison of both overall and individual antibiotic measurements between prescribers, general practices, hospitals, and countries. This is important to determine over time whether antibiotic consumption is increasing or decreasing, the ecological impact of antimicrobial prescribing at local, regional, and national levels, and whether the levels of specific agents are justifiable on the basis of resistance or other policy decisions. Two multinational European studies have demonstrated that antibiotic prescribing of penicillins, cephalosporins, and macrolides in primary care is significantly correlated with resistance in *Streptococcus pneumoniae* [14,15]. In addition, a pooled meta-analysis demonstrated that bacteria of both the urinary and respiratory tracts were more than twice as likely to have resistance detected within 2 months of patients receiving an antibiotic than those in patients who were not treated with antibiotics [16]. Antibiotic prescribing within hospitals is also known to select for resistant organisms [17].

The timeline of resistance development

The relationship between the development of resistance and time follows a sigmoid distribution. This is illustrated in Figure 1.2 using data from the European surveillance system for third-generation cephalosporin resistance. This demonstrates that after a prolonged lag phase, Sweden, despite its best efforts in antibiotic prescribing, has started to see an increase from 0% to 5% resistance over the last 13 years. Both the UK and Greece have gone through rapid increases in resistance: in the UK from 1% to almost 15% third-generation resistance in 13 years and in Greece from 4% to 17% in the same period. There were more than ten times more community prescriptions of third-generation cephalosporins in Greece [in 2000, 6.7 defined daily doses per 1000 inhabitants per day (DID)] than the UK (0.8 DID) or Sweden (0.5 DID). There is no doubt that the influence of both hospital and community prescribing combined had an impact on resistance that emerged and spread.

Since 2010, despite knowledge and awareness of the issue, there have been continued increases in AMR. The emergence of carbapenem resistance in *Klebsiella* across Europe is particularly important. Almost all countries are now reporting carbapenem resistance that varies from rare sporadic cases to regional spread across countries [19]. This suggests that if carbapenem resistance acts in a similar manner as described for cephalosporin resistance almost all countries in Europe will have a substantial problem by 2020 to 2025. This is demonstrated with the maps of resistance in *Klebsiella pneumoniae* from EARS-Net in 2009 and 2013. In 2013, Italy, Romania, and Greece reported very high proportions of carbapenem resistance (20.5, 34.3, and 59.4%, respectively), resulting in minimal, and in some cases no, effective antibiotic treatment being available for bloodstream infections in critically ill patients (see Figure 1.3).

With few new antibiotic treatment agents in development, there are a limited number of antibiotic treatment options available to treat resistant bacteria causing human and animal infections. It is essential that prudent prescribing occurs in both humans and animals to maintain

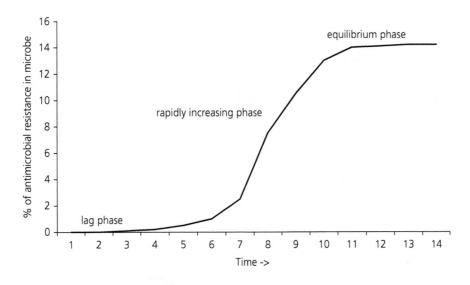

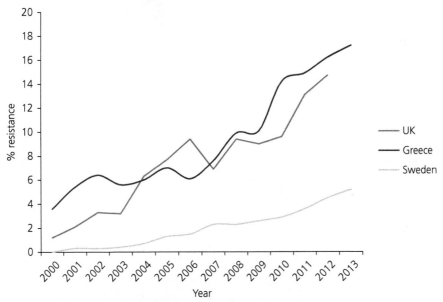

Figure 1.2 (a) The development of antimicrobial resistance over time [18] and (b) an example from Europe showing the proportion of *E. coli* resistant to third-generation cephalosporins in the UK, Sweden, and Greece, 2000–13 [19].

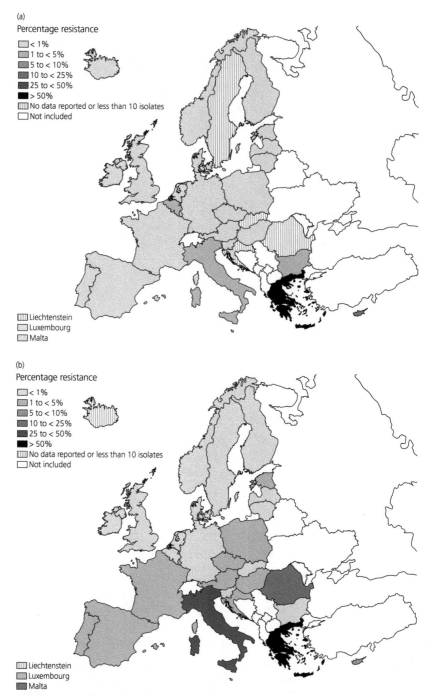

Figure 1.3 Carbapenem resistance in *Klebsiella pneumoniae* bloodstream infections in EU/EEA countries: (a) 2009 and (b) 2013 [19].

Reproduced with permission from European Centre for Disease Prevention and Control (ECDC), *Antimicrobial Resistance Interactive Database*, Copyright © ECDC, available from http://ecdc.europa.eu/en/healthtopics/antimicrobial_resistance/database/Pages/database.aspx, accessed November 2015.

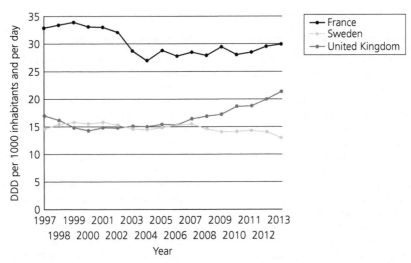

Figure 1.4 Trends in the consumption of antibiotics in the community from France, Sweden, and the UK, 1997–2013 [19].

Reproduced with permission from European Centre for Disease Prevention and Control (ECDC), *Antimicrobial Resistance Interactive Database*, Copyright © ECDC, available from http://ecdc.europa.eu/en/healthtopics/antimicrobial_resistance/database/Pages/database.aspx, accessed November 2015.

effectiveness of the antibiotics that are considered critically important to human health. It is therefore essential to understand how antibiotics are used and evaluate how prescribing can be optimized in human and veterinary medicine to limit the development of resistance. Antibiotic use continues to increase in many European countries; Figure 1.4 highlights three different patterns of community antibiotic consumption. While there are no international or national standards on the appropriate level of antibiotic consumption for each population, Sweden, which has the lowest consumption in Europe, is aiming to reduce consumption by at least a further 25% by 2020. In 2015, England introduced prescribing quality measures with the aim of reducing total antibiotic prescriptions in primary and secondary care.

Solutions to antimicrobial resistance

AMR control and antimicrobial development

AMR is a natural phenomenon that cannot be eliminated, but the development and spread of AMR can be slowed. The following approaches are key to the control of AMR: infection prevention and control, vaccination, antimicrobial stewardship, public and practitioner education, and a unified approach across human and animal health (commonly called 'one health').

There are two main methods for trying to control AMR: decrease the selection pressure of antimicrobials to prevent the selection of resistance and/or reduce the transmission of resistant organisms or the genetic determinants of resistance to prevent infection of other individuals. Examples of both of these approaches are outlined in Table 1.1.

Leadership, both political and clinical, across all countries will be required to stimulate key actions. The launch of the WHO global action plan will assist this, though it needs to be coupled with action on the ground through improved AMR surveillance, antimicrobial stewardship, better diagnostics, and effective infection prevention and control. Coupled with this, new antibiotics and clinical trials are required to determine the best drugs, treatment durations, and combinations for

Table 1.1 Measures to control AMR

Decrease selection pressure of antibiotics	Reduce transmission of AMR
1. Education of prescribers (both doctors and non-medical prescribers), pharmacists and nurses	1. Hand decontamination according to the WHO guidance
2. Prescriber audit and feedback	2. Environmental and equipment cleaning and decontamination especially in hospital
3. Antimicrobial restriction policies	3. Effective use of isolation rooms in hospitals and increased isolation rooms in new-builds and renovations
4. Antibiotic formulary restriction of key antibiotics of medical importance	
5. Limit duration of antibiotic prescription to the shortest possible	4. Decolonization of infected patients, where possible
6. Ensure that appropriate pharmacokinetic and pharmacodynamics measures are considered for each prescription	5. Improved detection of infected or colonized patients with rapid, timely and cost-effective laboratory diagnostics
7. Improve vaccinations to prevent infections and the need for antibiotics	6. Appropriate screening of hospital admissions for multidrug-resistant bacteria
8. Prevent infections developing through the use of technologies, e.g. silver-impregnated catheters	7. Sewage control in hospitals and the community
	8. Rapid control of outbreaks
	9. Recognition of high-risk health tourism
9. Electronic computer decision support	10. National and international surveillance to allow the detection and communication of emerging threats
10. Decrease use in animals, through effective animal biosafety and vaccination	

both multidrug-resistant infections and the key syndromes that contribute to AMR morbidity and mortality in individual patients.

The recent O'Neill report has highlighted that a new commercial model is required to encourage improved research and development of antibiotics [20]. Currently, commercial return on a new antibiotic is uncertain because clinicians and policy makers will want that antimicrobial to remain on the shelf to be used only in certain restricted conditions, often meaning that widespread use does not occur until close to the end of the life of the patent. One of the suggestions is to develop a global organization with lump sum payment on the development of a new antimicrobial that meets certain requirements. This would break the link between profitability of a drug and the volume of sales. Another suggestion is a global AMR innovation fund to allow 'blue-sky' thinking and innovative research, with Big Pharma investing in such a fund for 'enlightened self-interest'. Finally, there should be reduced barriers and improved efficiency for research and clinical trials, while maintaining patient safety.

Until new models for antimicrobial development are enacted new antimicrobials will remain in poor supply, and every prescriber must be required to improve antibiotic stewardship by every possible means.

References

1 De Kraker ME, Davey PG, Grundmann H; BURDEN Study Group. Mortality and hospital stay associated with resistant *Staphylococcus aureus* and *Escherichia coli* bacteremia: estimating the burden of antibiotic resistance in Europe. *PLoS Med* 2011;8:e1001104.

2 Abernethy JK, Johnson AP, Guy R, Hinton N, Sheridan EA, Hope RJ. Thirty day all-cause mortality in patients with *Escherichia coli* bacteraemia in England. *Clin Microbiol Infect* 2015;21:251.e1–8.

3 Liu L, Oza S, Hogan D, Perin J, Rudan I, Lawn JE, et al. Global, regional, and national causes of child mortality in 2000–13, with projections to inform post-2015 priorities: an updated systematic analysis. *Lancet* 2015;385:430–40.

4 *Antimicrobial resistance: tackling a crisis for the health and wealth of nations*. The review on antimicrobial resistance chaired by Jim O'Neill. December 2014. Available at: http://www.jpiamr.eu/wp-content/uploads/2014/12/AMR-Review-Paper-Tackling-a-crisis-for-the-health-and-wealth-of-nations_1-2.pdf

5 *Annual report of the Chief Medical Officer 2011: volume two*. Infections and the rise of antimicrobial resistance. Available at: https://www.gov.uk/government/publications/chief-medical-officer-annual-report-volume-2

6 **Department of Health**. *UK five year antimicrobial resistance strategy 2013 to 2018*. 2013. Available at: https://www.gov.uk/government/uploads/system/uploads/attachment_data/file/244058/20130902_UK_5_year_AMR_strategy.pdf

7 The Global Health Security Agenda. Available at: http://www.globalhealth.gov/global-health-topics/global-health-security/ghsagenda.html

8 **Kuenzli E, Jaeger VK, Frei R, Neumayr A, DeCrom S, Haller S, et al.** High colonization rates of extended-spectrum β-lactamase (ESBL)-producing *Escherichia coli* in Swiss travellers to South Asia—a prospective observational multicentre cohort study looking at epidemiology, microbiology and risk factors. *BMC Infect Dis* 2014;**14**:528.

9 *ESBLs: a threat to human and animal health?* Report by the Joint Working Group of DARC and ARHAI. 2012. Available at: https://www.gov.uk/government/publications/esbls-a-threat-to-human-and-animal-health

10 *English National Point Prevalence Survey on healthcare-associated infection and antimicrobial use: 2011*. Available at: https://www.gov.uk/government/publications/healthcare-associated-infections-hcai-point-prevalence-survey-england

11 **Cotta MO, Robertson MS, Upjohn LM, Marshall C, Liew D, Buising KL.** Using periodic point-prevalence surveys to assess appropriateness of antimicrobial prescribing in Australian private hospitals. *Intern Med J* 2014;**44**:240–6.

12 **Artoisenet C, Ausselet N, Delaere B, Spinewine A.** Evaluation of the appropriateness of intravenous amoxicillin/clavulanate prescription in a teaching hospital. *Acta Clin Belg* 2013;**68**:81–6.

13 **Scottish Antimicrobial Prescribing Group.** *Primary care prescribing indicators. Annual report 2013–14.* Available at: https://isdscotland.scot.nhs.uk/Health-Topics/Prescribing-and-Medicines/Publications/2014-10-14/2014-10-14-SAPG-Primary-Care-PI-2013-14-Report.pdf

14 **Bronzwaer SL, Cars O, Buchholz U, Molstad S, Goettsch W, Veldhuijzen IK et al.** A European study on the relationship between antimicrobial use and antimicrobial resistance. *Emerg Infect Dis* 2002;**8**:278–82.

15 **Goossens H, Ferech M, Vander SR, Elseviers M.** Outpatient antibiotic use in Europe and association with resistance: a cross-national database study. *Lancet* 2005;**365**:579–87.

16 **Costelloe C, Metcalfe C, Lovering A, Mant D, Hay AD.** Effect of antibiotic prescribing in primary care on antimicrobial resistance in individual patients: systematic review and meta-analysis. *Br Med J* 2010;**340**:c2096.

17 **Tacconelli E, De AG, Cataldo MA, Mantengoli E, Spanu T, Pan A et al.** Antibiotic usage and risk of colonization and infection with antibiotic-resistant bacteria: a hospital population-based study. *Antimicrob Agents Chemother* 2009;**53**:4264–69.

18 **Smith RD, Coast J, Millar MR, Wilton P, Karcher AM.** *Interventions against antimicrobial resistance: a review of the literature and exploration of modelling cost-effectiveness.* Global Forum for Health Research, September 2001. Available at: http://announcementsfiles.cohred.org/gfhr_pub/assoc/s14820e/s14820e.pdf

19 **European Centre for Disease Prevention and Control.** Antimicrobial Resistance Interactive Database (EARS-net). Available at: http://ecdc.europa.eu/en/healthtopics/antimicrobial_resistance/database/Pages/database.aspx (last accessed 6 June 2015).

20 *Securing new drugs for future generations: the pipeline of antibiotics*. The Review on Antimicrobial Resistance. Chaired by Jim O'Neill. London. 2015. Available at: http://amr-review.org/Publications

Chapter 2

What are the principles and goals of antimicrobial stewardship?

Fiona Robb and Andrew Seaton

Introduction to the principles and goals of antimicrobial stewardship

The aim of antimicrobial therapy is to effect cure of infection or, in some circumstances, to prevent infection. Benefits, from cure of life-threatening microbial infections to a vital supporting role in many modern medical advances, have occurred in the 'blink of an eye' relative to human history and have been followed apace by the development and recognition of antimicrobial resistance (AMR). In Alexander Fleming's 1945 Nobel Lecture [1] he warned:

> The time may come when penicillin may be bought by anyone in the shops. Then there is the danger that the ignorant may easily under-dose himself and by exposing his microbes to non-lethal quantities of the drug make them resistant.

Despite Fleming's warnings, 70 years later the World Health Organization (WHO) reported [2]:

> In most countries, antibiotics can be purchased in markets, shops, pharmacies or over the internet without prescription or involvement of a health professional or veterinarian. Poor quality medical and veterinary products are widespread, and often contain low concentrations of active ingredients, encouraging emergence of resistant microbes.

AMR has developed, to a degree, to all available antimicrobials. Combined with a drought of novel therapies, there are increasing limitations on treatment options for resistant infections.

Other important 'collateral' or unwanted effects of antimicrobials include the 'unseen' alterations of the gut flora, a critical step in susceptibility to *Clostridium difficile* acquisition and infection (CDI).

Together, AMR and CDI are of major importance, particularly in settings where broad-spectrum prescribing is combined with susceptible, vulnerable patient populations. Resultant healthcare-associated infections (HCAI), estimated to occur in 4.9% of patients in acute hospital care settings in Europe, highlight the fundamental importance of antimicrobial prescribing in modern healthcare [3].

Observation of international differences in resistance, correlating with the volume of antimicrobials consumed in different populations, gives hope that antimicrobial control may be key to controlling resistance. In Nordic countries, where prescribing of antimicrobials is restrictive and regulated, rates of methicillin-resistant *Staphylococcus aureus* (MRSA) are low (<5%) compared with southern Europe where antimicrobial regulation has been less evident and MRSA rates are high (25–50%) [4]. There are historical examples where strict antibiotic restrictions have been associated with precipitous reductions in certain infections [5].

Improving the utilization of existing antimicrobials has been central to national AMR strategies. The 'UK five year antimicrobial resistance strategy 2013 to 2018' [6] emphasizes the importance of strategies to improve the quality and safety of prescribing, the conservation of currently available agents with increased surveillance of antimicrobial utilization and resistance patterns in conjunction with implementation of improved infection control practices, and the development of new diagnostics and antimicrobials. The UK strategy is complemented by other resources from UK administrations including the 'Scottish management of antimicrobial resistance action plan 2014–18' (ScotMARAP 2) [7], which includes division of responsibility through health structures from government to individual healthcare professionals. The 2015 WHO global action plan on resistance sets out five strategic objectives including improvement of the utilization of antimicrobials [2].

What is antimicrobial stewardship?

Antimicrobial stewardship (AMS) is a coordinated, quality improvement strategy designed to encourage the appropriate use of antimicrobial agents to optimize clinical outcomes while minimizing collateral antimicrobial effects. Collateral effects are primarily AMR and CDI but also include any other adverse antimicrobial event. AMS promotes prudent, effective prescribing through optimization of antimicrobial selection, dosage, duration of treatment, and route of administration [8].

An AMS programme (ASP) is one empowered by an organization to deliver AMS on its behalf. It encompasses both clinical leadership in prescribing and corporate responsibility for prescribing practice, including strategy, surveillance of antimicrobial use, and education relating to antimicrobial therapy. Availability of prescribing and resistance data and an understanding of prescribing culture and practice are fundamental to inform interventions, guidance, and educational activities (Box 2.1). Traditionally ASPs have focused on hospital-based prescribing, where the use of broad-spectrum antibiotics is most prevalent and infections most severe.

An example of the principles and framework for AMS are outlined in the 2005 document 'Antimicrobial prescribing policy and practice in Scotland: recommendations for good antimicrobial

Box 2.1 Key requirements and functions of an antimicrobial stewardship programme

An ASP should:

1 Deliver the national antibiotic agenda locally, optimize antibiotic prescribing, and with infection prevention control teams contribute towards reduction in antibiotic resistance and healthcare-associated infections including CDI.

2 Receive support from clinical and managerial leadership who are accountable for the ASP outcomes.

3 Develop and implement appropriate educational packages for all healthcare professionals to improve knowledge of antibiotics and to support the ASP interventions.

4 Promote adherence to recommended good antibiotic prescribing practices.

5 Develop and survey standard datasets of antibiotic usage and antimicrobial resistance.

6 Audit and feed back the results of any new intervention and interpreted surveillance data to key stakeholders.

7 Assess adherence to antibiotic guidelines and progress towards national antibiotic targets through the introduction of performance indications.

8 Have flexibility to respond acutely to emerging challenges including collaborating with IPC teams during HCAI outbreaks where antibiotic prescribing may be implicated.

practice in acute hospitals' [9] in which key recommendations are made regarding the delivery of good antimicrobial practice in acute hospitals. These include recommendations for training, audit, and performance indicators as well as the definition and development of antimicrobial management structures, including the formation of multidisciplinary antimicrobial management teams (AMTs), who have responsibility, and accountability. In 2008, the Scottish Government extended the remit of ASPs by directing all health boards to appoint AMTs with responsibility for both hospital and community-based prescribing in response to increasing concerns regarding CDI [10].

The antimicrobial management team

At the heart of an ASP is its interdisciplinary AMT [8,9]. Expertise within the team should encompass therapeutics, AMR, diagnostics, and clinical infection management. Typically the team should comprise medical infection specialists, clinicians, and antimicrobial pharmacists with close links to laboratory diagnostics, infection prevention control teams, and information technology systems. Antimicrobial pharmacists are key individuals who support and direct AMS activities, and in the UK their expertise is supported by an expert professional curriculum [11]. While the AMT is responsible for stewardship strategy it should be informed by representation of key stakeholders and clinical experts both internal and external to the organization. These should include general practitioners and pharmacy prescribing advisers, hospital-based clinicians representing major prescribing specialities (e.g. medicine, surgery, intensive care, haemato-oncology, and paediatrics), specialist hospital-based pharmacists, nursing professionals, the infection prevention and control (IPC) team, and patient safety teams.

ASPs are unique within healthcare, lying between two traditionally separate streams of governance, namely IPC and therapeutics. It is important therefore that the AMT communicates through both channels, sharing intelligence regarding prescribing practice and AMR (and other consequences of prescribing) and keeping both abreast of developments and interventions. In order to ensure implementation of strategy, guidance, and quality improvement it is essential that there are lines of communication between the AMT and senior healthcare management including speciality clinical leaders. It is also important that the AMT works with clinical governance and risk management teams to ensure the implementation of safe and effective antibiotic guidelines. These relationships support monitoring for outcomes, including unintended consequences, and ensure that measures to resolve issues and implement improvement processes are in place (Figure 2.1).

Specific aims of an antimicrobial stewardship programme

An ASP aims to improve antibiotic prescribing, minimize harm, reduce antibiotic resistance and HCAI, and promote cost-effective prescribing. These aims are supported by a series of primary objectives, or 'drivers', including robust stewardship infrastructure, improved education on antibiotics, introduction of good antimicrobial prescribing practices, surveillance of antimicrobial usage and resistance patterns, audit and feedback of antimicrobial policies, and application of quality performance indicators. Each intervention is underpinned by the prudent antimicrobial prescribing ethos 'the right drug at the right time at the right dose for the right duration' [8].

Primary objectives may be further broken down by 'secondary drivers' or planned projects and activities designed to achieve the primary objectives and overall aims. Activities include development of infection management and surgical prophylaxis guidelines, development of education packages, and collaborative working with IPC teams. Interventions are therefore measurable, providing an opportunity to track progress towards achieving the overall aims. It is important that

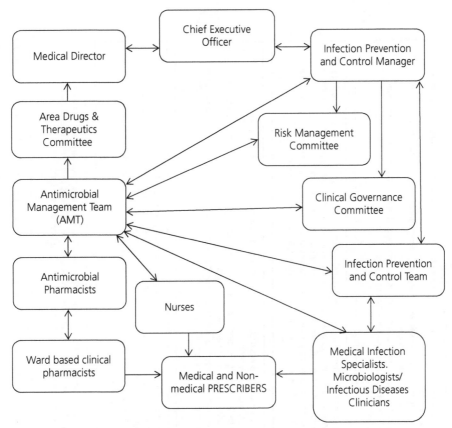

Figure 2.1 Key relationships in an ASP.

this plan is dynamic and adjustable to address local and national ASP priorities. An example of an antimicrobial stewardship driver diagram used within ScotMARAP 2 [2] and adapted from the Centers for Disease Control and Prevention and Public Health Institute in the USA [12] is shown in Figure 2.2. The driver diagram includes key ASP themes, two of which are described below together with the need for leadership. The remaining themes are described in other chapters of this book.

Education

To ensure the continued sustainability of any ASP it is important to provide a solid foundation of knowledge about antimicrobial stewardship and infection prevention and control tailored appropriately for all healthcare professionals. Embedding the principles of antimicrobial stewardship and adherence to infection guidelines within medical, pharmacy, and nursing school curricula is fundamental to this end. Of particular importance for medical prescribers as they transition from student to practitioner is practical induction into prudent prescribing practice. For post-graduates the development of various multidisciplinary educational resources and initiatives, including case-based learning, on-line learning modules, electronic updates, webinars, and 'bedside learning' via infection specialist-led antimicrobial rounds, is important. Continuous feedback on prescribing practice and involvement in quality improvement programmes is of particular value in reinforcing

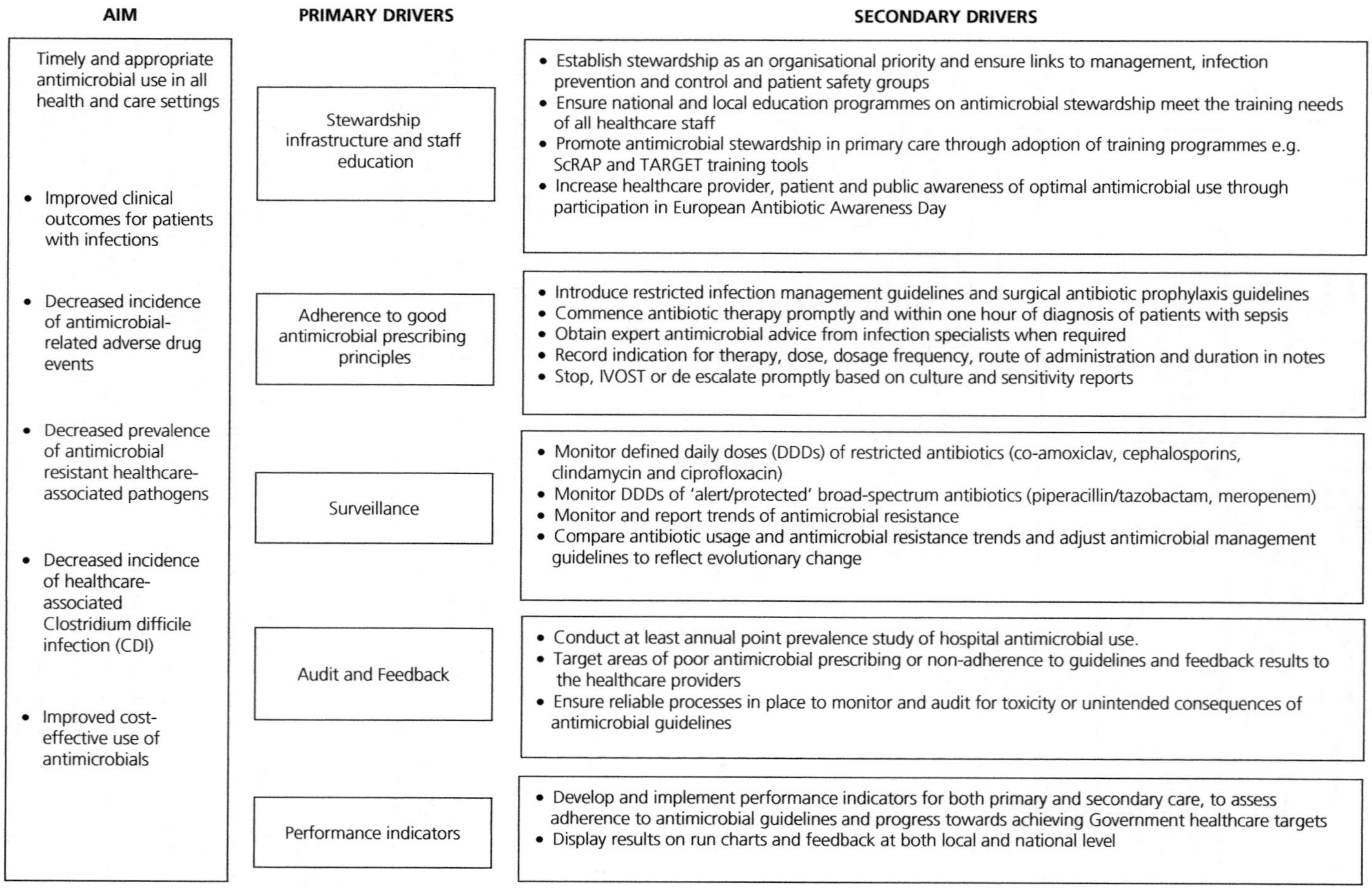

AIM

- Timely and appropriate antimicrobial use in all health and care settings
- Improved clinical outcomes for patients with infections

- Decreased incidence of antimicrobial-related adverse drug events

- Decreased prevalence of antimicrobial resistant healthcare-associated pathogens
- Decreased incidence of healthcare-associated Clostridium difficile infection (CDI)
- Improved cost-effective use of antimicrobials

PRIMARY DRIVERS

Stewardship infrastructure and staff education

Adherence to good antimicrobial prescribing principles

Surveillance

Audit and Feedback

Performance indicators

SECONDARY DRIVERS

- Establish stewardship as an organisational priority and ensure links to management, infection prevention and control and patient safety groups
- Ensure national and local education programmes on antimicrobial stewardship meet the training needs of all healthcare staff
- Promote antimicrobial stewardship in primary care through adoption of training programmes e.g. ScRAP and TARGET training tools
- Increase healthcare provider, patient and public awareness of optimal antimicrobial use through participation in European Antibiotic Awareness Day

- Introduce restricted infection management guidelines and surgical antibiotic prophylaxis guidelines
- Commence antibiotic therapy promptly and within one hour of diagnosis of patients with sepsis
- Obtain expert antimicrobial advice from infection specialists when required
- Record indication for therapy, dose, dosage frequency, route of administration and duration in notes
- Stop, IVOST or de escalate promptly based on culture and sensitivity reports

- Monitor defined daily doses (DDDs) of restricted antibiotics (co-amoxiclav, cephalosporins, clindamycin and ciprofloxacin)
- Monitor DDDs of 'alert/protected' broad-spectrum antibiotics (piperacillin/tazobactam, meropenem)
- Monitor and report trends of antimicrobial resistance
- Compare antibiotic usage and antimicrobial resistance trends and adjust antimicrobial management guidelines to reflect evolutionary change

- Conduct at least annual point prevalence study of hospital antimicrobial use.
- Target areas of poor antimicrobial prescribing or non-adherence to guidelines and feedback results to the healthcare providers
- Ensure reliable processes in place to monitor and audit for toxicity or unintended consequences of antimicrobial guidelines

- Develop and implement performance indicators for both primary and secondary care, to assess adherence to antimicrobial guidelines and progress towards achieving Government healthcare targets
- Display results on run charts and feedback at both local and national level

Figure 2.2 An example of an antimicrobial stewardship driver diagram (IVOST, intravenous to oral antibiotic switch therapy).

Source: data from World Health Organization, *Antimicrobial resistance draft global action plan on antimicrobial resistance*, Sixty-Eighth World Health Assembly, 27th March 2015, Copyright © WHO 2015, available from http://apps.who.int/gb/ebwha/pdf_files/WHA68/A68_20-en.pdf?ua=1; and Institute for Health Improvement, *CDC Antimicrobial Stewardship Driver Diagram*, available from http://www.cdc.gov/getsmart/healthcare/pdfs/Antibiotic_Stewardship_Driver_Diagram_10_30_12.pdf good prescribing practice, whilst demonstration of learning attainment can be used for professional appraisal and revalidation.

In UK primary care, interactive, case-based antimicrobial education tools include TARGET ('treat antibiotics responsibly, guidance, education, tools') [13], which is supported by the Royal College of General Practitioners, and the Scottish reduction in AMR (ScRAP) programme [14].

The Professional Education sub-group of the Expert Advisory Committee on AMR and Healthcare Associated Infections and Public Health England have developed a progressive competency framework entitled 'Antimicrobial prescribing and stewardship competencies' designed for prescribers across primary and secondary care [15]. This should complement continuous professional development relating to antibiotics for prescribers at all levels, regardless of speciality. Similarly, NHS Education for Scotland has developed an educational package supporting stewardship among nurses [16].

Raising awareness and educating users of the healthcare system is clearly important. The annual European Antibiotic Awareness Day is a public health initiative that provides the opportunity to focus on ASPs by engaging all healthcare staff and members of the public [17].

Quality performance targets

In the UK, performance indicators support the delivery of national and local health priorities. These include targets supporting and evaluating adherence to ASPs. Prescribing indicators are valuable in giving recognition and priority to ASPs and drive improvements in practice supporting reduction in HCAI and AMR.

In Scotland, hospital-based indicators include empirical antibiotic prescribing targets (compliance with policy and rationale for treatment recorded in ≥ 95% of cases) and surgical prophylaxis (a single dose of a policy-compliant antibiotic given in elective surgery in ≥ 95% of cases) [18]. Local feedback by AMTs to clinicians drives improvement locally, while national comparisons can also be made. Local clinician involvement engages and promotes improvement in practice.

In primary care in Scotland, seasonal variation in fluoroquinolone prescribing of less than 5% was selected as a prescribing indicator to reduce observed inappropriate prescribing for respiratory tract infections in winter. Educational activities, prescribing prompts, and feedback through prescribing advisors supported changes in practice and improvements were observed [19]. Subsequently an indicator to reduce total antibiotic usage was adopted with a focus on shorter-course therapy and the avoidance of unnecessary prescribing for viral infections. The measure is items dispensed/1000 days with a target of ≥ 50% GP practices to achieve/make significant movement towards the lower 25th percentile of antibiotic prescribers [19]. This target is supported by the ScRAP toolkit [14].

The importance of national leadership in antimicrobial stewardship

To enable delivery of a safe and effective ASP there must be clinical leadership, engagement with prescribers and key stakeholders, management support, and adequate funding. National prioritization is essential to support local practice. ASPs now have a global priority and are embedded in health strategy in many countries, including much of Europe, Australasia, and the USA. There are great challenges in delivering ASP in countries with poor health infrastructure or where there are cultural barriers towards restricting individual prescribing practice. Locally sensitive solutions should be supported by evidence and expertise from countries with advanced stewardship practice.

Whilst long-term global strategies are required, application of an ASP that engages commitment from key stakeholders at both national and local level makes it possible to significantly improve patient safety and the quality of antimicrobial prescribing for potentially large populations of patients.

References

1 **Fleming A.** Penicillin. Nobel Lecture, December 11, 1945. http://www.nobelprize.org/nobel_prizes/medicine/laureates/1945/fleming-lecture.pdf

2 **World Health Organization.** Antimicrobial resistance. Draft global action plan on antimicrobial resistance. Sixty-Eighth World Health Assembly, 27 March 2015. http://apps.who.int/gb/ebwha/pdf_files/WHA68/A68_20-en.pdf?ua=1

3 **Zarb P, Amadeo B, Muller A, Drapier N, Vankerckhoven V, Davey P, et al.** Identification of targets for quality improvement in antimicrobial prescribing: the web-based ESAC Point Prevalence Survey 2009. *J Antimicrob Chemother* 2011;**66**:443–49.

4 **European Centre for Disease Prevention and Control.** Proportion of methicillin resistant *Staphylococcus aureus* (MRSA) isolates in participating countries in 2013. http://ecdc.europa.eu/en/healthtopics/antimicrobial_resistance/database/Pages/map_reports.aspx

5 **Price DJE, Sleigh DJ.** Control of infection due to *Klebsiella aerogenes* in a neurosurgical unit by withdrawal of all antibiotics. *Lancet* 1970;**296**:1213–15.

6 **Department of Health.** *UK five year antimicrobial resistance strategy 2013 to 2018.* 2013. Available at: https://www.gov.uk/government/uploads/system/uploads/attachment_data/file/244058/20130902_UK_5_year_AMR_strategy.pdf (accessed 2 June 2014).

7 **The Scottish Government.** *Scottish management of antimicrobial resistance action plan 2014–18 (ScotMARAP 2).* 2014. Available at: http://www.gov.scot/Resource/0045/00456736.pdf

8 **Dellit TH, Owens RC, McGowan JE et al.** Infectious Diseases Society of America and the Society for Healthcare Epidemiology of America guidelines for developing an institutional program to enhance antimicrobial stewardship. *Clin Infect Dis* 2007;**44**:159–77.

9 **Scottish Antimicrobial Prescribing Policy and Practice Group.** *Antimicrobial prescribing policy and practice in Scotland: recommendations for good antimicrobial practice in acute hospitals.* September 2005. Available at: http://www.gov.scot/Publications/2005/09/02132609/26114

10 **The Scottish Government.** *Prudent antimicrobial prescribing: the Scottish action plan for managing antibiotic resistance and reducing antibiotic related* Clostridium difficile *associated disease.* Available at: http://www.sehd.scot.nhs.uk/mels/CEL2008_30.pdf

11 **Sneddon J, Gilchrist M, Wickens H.** Development of an expert curriculum for antimicrobial pharmacists in the UK. *J Antimicrob Chemother* 2015;**70**:1277–80.

12 **Institute for Health Improvement/CDC.** Antimicrobial stewardship driver diagram. Available at: http://www.cdc.gov/getsmart/healthcare/pdfs/Antibiotic_Stewardship_Driver_Diagram_10_30_12.pdf

13 **Royal College of General Practitioners.** TARGET antibiotics toolkit. Available at: http://www.rcgp.org.uk/TARGETantibiotics

14 **NHS Education for Scotland.** Scottish reduction in antimicrobial prescribing (ScRAP) programme. 2013. Available at: http://www.nes.scot.nhs.uk/education-and-training/by-discipline/pharmacy/about-nes-pharmacy/educational-resources/resources-by-topic/infectious-diseases/antibiotics/scottish-reduction-in-antimicrobial-prescribing-%28scrap%29-programme.aspx

15 **Department of Health Expert Advisory Committee on Antimicrobial Resistance and Healthcare Associated Infection (ARHAI) and Public Health England.** *Antimicrobial prescribing and stewardship competencies.* 2013. Available at: http://www.his.org.uk/files/2413/8122/1363/PHE_Antimicorbial_Prescribing_and_Stewardship_Competencies.pdf

16 **NHS Education for Scotland.** Antimicrobial resistance and stewardship. Educational resource to support antimicrobial prescribing, resistance and stewardship within NHS Scotland. Available

at: http://www.nes.scot.nhs.uk/education-and-training/by-theme-initiative/healthcare-associated-infections/educational-programmes/antimicrobial-resistance-and-stewardship.aspx

17 **Public Health England.** Antibiotic awareness resources. Available at: https://www.gov.uk/government/collections/european-antibiotic-awareness-day-resources

18 **Nathwani D, Sneddon J, Malcolm W, Wiuff C, Patton A, Hurding S et al.** Scottish Antimicrobial Prescribing Group (SAPG): development and impact of the Scottish National Antimicrobial Stewardship Programme. *IntJ Antimicrob Agents* 2011;**38**:16–26.

19 **Scottish Antimicrobial Prescribing Group**. *Primary care prescribing indicators. Annual report 2013–14.* October 2014. Available at: http://www.scottishmedicines.org.uk/SAPG/News/2014-10-14-SAPG-Primary-Care-PI-2013-14-Report.pdf

Chapter 3

Managing behaviours: social, cultural, and psychological aspects of antibiotic prescribing and use

Esmita Charani and Gabriel Birgand

Introduction to managing behaviours

The association between antibiotic consumption and the emergence of antibiotic resistance is well established, and yet antibiotic prescribing remains suboptimal [1]. To address this issue, governments and organizations implement policy- and practice-based interventions [2]. This approach assumes that the behaviour of prescribers is congruent with these interventions. The unintended consequence of antibiotic use, the emergence of resistance, is intangible at the point of antibiotic prescribing and consumption and remains difficult to translate into prescribing policy. The social, cultural, and environmental factors that might affect behaviour are rarely taken into account when developing interventions [3]. This may well be one of the reasons why it remains a challenge to optimize antibiotic prescribing. Theoretical frameworks from psychology and social sciences that address the issues of how to change behaviour and sustain such change over time remain underused. Antibiotic stewardship programmes need to incorporate in their design an understanding of the cognitive biases that underpin prescribing behaviour.

Most interventions targeting antibiotic prescribing in secondary care have at their core the intention to change prescribing behaviours. However, very few published studies have attempted to incorporate social science research into their methods [4]. Studies that have tried to apply the social and human sciences to research in antibiotic stewardship have highlighted the important influence of underlying cultures and etiquette on antibiotic prescribing behaviours [5].

This chapter invites the reader to reflect on the significance of the social, cultural, and psychological determinants of antibiotic prescribing behaviours. It will describe why the social sciences cannot be overlooked in antibiotic stewardship, and provide examples of how to apply these principles in practice using real cases, with emphasis on strategies for changing behaviour.

The multifaceted aspect of antibiotic prescribing

Antibiotics have been instrumental in saving millions of lives by treating infectious diseases that were a major cause of death until the early decades of the twentieth century. It can be argued that they have made the single most significant contribution to public health. In their early use, antibiotics were ferociously promoted as a 'cure-all' intervention. Thus, antibiotics became a common matter-of-fact solution available to any prescriber. A prescription for an antibiotic is viewed as a trivial commodity that provides a clear individual benefit to patients without any major side effects. This perception of antibiotics is now embedded in medical and social culture. However, this is a deep-rooted misconception. The excessive and indiscriminate use of these so-called miracle drugs has led to the emergence and dissemination of resistant organisms that render antibiotics ineffective [6]. The uncontrolled use of antibiotics leads to collateral damage, not only putting at risk the patient being treated but also jeopardizing the future treatment of other patients.

Medical education has followed a very specific path, with students and doctors being trained through pathways to cure patients using the most effective strategy. This education policy is now deeply entrenched in medical culture. Through the boom in information technology, patients are also exposed to medical practices and so-called knowledge that is unchecked, unverified, and sometimes inaccurate. Their perceptions and expectations put an external pressure on the prescriber in the commercial context of health. Thus, the prescription of antibiotics is the result of a complex deliberative process balancing short-term benefits to the patient with the negative medium- to long-term effects on bacterial ecology, with selection of multi-drug resistant (MDR) organisms.

This conflict between individual benefit clearly tangible to the prescriber and the patient and insidious and invisible collateral damage introduces a strong psychological component into the complex process of antibiotic prescribing and consumption.

Evidence from social science—why we need to address culture

Two examples of the use of social science in other fields

The limited application of key theories of behaviour change in antibiotic interventions contrasts with other areas that have demonstrated the success of providing goal-setting, feedback, and action planning in changing the behaviour of health professionals in hospitals.

The first example is intervention to improve hand hygiene, with the successful use of 'actionable feedback' [7]. This model emphasizes that feedback should be timely, individualized, non-punitive, and customized. Providing real-time feedback for antibiotic use requires the collection and analysis of numerous data elements to examine trends in use. For antibiotic stewardship, it may be more challenging to assign individual responsibility for actions than it is for simpler behavioural targets such as hand hygiene. In secondary care, clinicians view antibiotic prescribing as a shared responsibility between practitioners who assess a patient's clinical signs and laboratory data over the course of his or her illness [8].

A second example of quality improvement through actionable feedback is the Michigan intensive care unit (ICU) project [9] which achieved a significant reduction in central line-associated bloodstream infections. This successful intervention was based on the use of checklists that reminded participants about the care bundle elements to be implemented. The checklist may have stimulated a culture change, increasing safety as a priority for the participating clinical teams. A detailed ethnographic study following the implementation of the same checklist in the UK revealed marked differences between the few ICUs that achieved reduction in central line bloodstream infections versus the majority that did not [9]. In successful ICUs, data collection was embedded into the daily routine with reminders about important care processes and regular feedback and discussion of results. In contrast, in the unsuccessful ICUs information and decisions about infections were collected by external people responsible for delivery of the intervention. So the successful interventions were characterized by self-monitoring as well as by actionable feedback.

Cultural aspects

The variation in antibiotic consumption across countries, hospitals, and specialities underscores the potential influence of culture on antibiotic prescribing [10]. People hold different ideas about health, the causes of disease, labelling of illness, and treatment modalities. These ideas shape both the expectations and the behaviour of healthcare professionals. Furthermore, such ideas are shaped and reinforced thorough local prevailing cultures, for example within specialities.

Concepts of 'uncertainty avoidance' (i.e. an unwillingness to accept uncertainty and risks) and 'power distance' (i.e. a willingness to accept that power is unevenly distributed) have been described as the reasons for cultural influences [11]. Antibiotics have a defensive function: the prescriber and the patient aim for certainty.

The culture-specific way that people deal with authority is important in explaining differences in antibiotic use and the part played by uncertainty avoidance. At the country scale, egalitarian societies (the Netherlands, the UK, and Scandinavian countries) consume fewer antibiotics than hierarchical societies (France, Italy, Spain, Portugal, and Greece) [12]. In hierarchical societies antibiotics may provide the healthcare professional with therapeutic power. These differences in use coincide with differences in religion [13].

Contextual aspects

Physicians within hospitals fail to use antibiotics appropriately in the presence of an internal obstacle that has a cognitive (knowledge) or affective (attitude) component, or in the presence of an external obstacle (organizational, social, political, or economic) that restricts professionals' abilities.

External organizational obstacles influence the timeliness of antibiotic administration, i.e. laboratory results or lack of antibiotics. In a Cochrane review, 27 studies used organizational strategies (i.e. selective reporting of laboratory susceptibilities, formulary restriction) and three studies of structural organizational strategies (quality monitoring mechanisms) to improve prescribing [14]. However, the degree to which these various policies are used differs greatly between hospitals.

Different hospital disciplines are usually involved in antibiotic prescribing (e.g. clinicians, nurses, pharmacists, microbiologists) requiring important ingredients (e.g. care coordination, collaboration and communication between professionals, teamwork, and care logistics). This multi-professional care delivery system enhances clinical expertise and provides better care due to the insights of different bodies of knowledge and a wider range of skills.

Behavioural aspects

The gap between the care recommended in guidelines and the care provided varies across and within organizations [15]. Many individual characteristics, such as the professional background or clinical experience of healthcare professionals, can influence antibiotic use or beliefs about antibiotic practice [16]. Disagreement with recommendations, lack of outcome expectancy, lack of self-efficacy expectations, and lack of motivation might all lead to suboptimal antibiotic use.

In-depth interviews with physicians indicate that perceived characteristics of a critical pathway (limited applicability, lack of flexibility to accommodate atypical clinical presentations, and perception of insufficient evidence to support recommendations), and the physician's need for local adaptation, influence adherence to that pathway [17].

Application of behaviour change to improve antibiotic prescribing

Behaviour change interventions

Interventions to improve antibiotic prescribing can be divided into three different categories (Table 3.1). Overall, restrictive interventions are more successful in the short term [14]. However, the overwhelming majority of studies provide minimal insight into the sustainability and unintended consequences of the interventions described. To be part of an effective and sustainable antibiotic stewardship programme, interventions should become a core component of patient safety programmes within healthcare systems [18]. Successful embedding of interventions into patient safety programmes requires a greater understanding of the prevailing systems and cultures in order that new interventions are integrated into existing decision architecture and pathways [19]. It is necessary to evaluate the differences in efficacy between various stewardship interventions and the impact of inclusion of behaviour change science into the development and implementation of interventions.

Essential points for the implementation of behaviour change techniques

Published studies have identified the elements of behaviour change interventions as goal setting, self-monitoring, feedback, and action planning.

Table 3.1 Categories of behaviour change interventions in antibiotic prescribing

Types of intervention	Example
Persuasive interventions	Distribution of educational material
	Educational meetings
	Local consensus processes
	Educational outreach visits
	Local opinion leaders
	Reminders provided verbally, on paper, or on computer
	Audit and feedback
Restrictive interventions: a change to the antibiotic formulary or policy implemented through an organizational change that restricts the freedom of prescribers to select some antibiotics	A compulsory order form (prescribers have to complete a form with clinical details to justify use of the restricted antibiotics)
	Expert approval (the prescription has to be approved by an infection specialist or by the head of department)
	Restriction by removal (removing restricted antibiotics from drug cupboards)
	Review and make change (the reviewer changes the prescription rather than giving health professionals either a verbal or written recommendation that they should change the prescription)
Structural interventions	Changing from paper to computerized records
	Rapid laboratory testing, computerized decision support systems
	Introduction or organization of quality monitoring mechanisms

Text extracts reproduced with permission from Davey P et al., 'Interventions to improve antibiotic prescribing practices for hospital inpatients (Review)', *Cochrane Database of Systematic Reviews 2013*, Issue 4. Art. No.: CD003543, Copyright © 2013 The Cochrane Collaboration. Published by John Wiley & Sons, Ltd.

The quality of delivery of goal-setting (e.g. specificity, clarity, timeliness, with/without encouragement) has been shown to be associated with the effectiveness of the technique when applied to smoking cessation [20]. When implementing behaviour change interventions, it is crucial to be in agreement with stakeholders on a goal defined in terms of the behaviour to be achieved or a positive outcome of wanted behaviour. In the literature, goals are generally poorly specified in interventions, with communication of threshold and timing to participants being implied rather than explicit [4,21].

Feedback could be defined as the monitoring needed to provide informative or evaluative feedback on performance of the behaviour (e.g. form, frequency, duration, intensity). Feedback alone is only moderately effective, but combining it with goal-setting and action planning is associated with significantly enhanced effectiveness of audit and feedback interventions [22]. Behaviour change is most likely if feedback about one's performance is accompanied by a comparison with a performance target and the provision of strategies to reduce discrepancies between one's target and one's actual performance [22]. Successful interventions include embedding data collection into the daily routine and reminders about important care processes, as well as by regular feedback and discussion of results. This type of intervention combines actionable feedback and self-monitoring [23]. Self-monitoring is the establishment of a method for the person to monitor and record their behaviour(s). As already noted, self-monitoring is usually more effective if it is combined with the provision of feedback, goal-setting, and action planning.

Action planning has been found to be an important technique in many behaviour change studies (of obesity or smoking cessation) [24]. It could be defined as the prompt detailed planning of performance of the behaviour (which must include at least one of context, frequency, duration, and intensity). An example of action planning is as follows: each clinical team has an identified coordinator who observes practices at both individual and group level and identifies a clear alternative strategy from the outset should the predefined targets not be met. The intervention can include rewards for achieving the target behaviour (e.g. a certificate that could be filed for use in professional development appraisal). A dose effect for action planning has been described by an increase in effectiveness with the number of action plans that are written [25].

Antibiotic stewardship—the key stakeholders

The key to successful teamwork requires an understanding of the champions and opinion leaders within clinical groups, who can then become engaged in stewardship activities and be encouraged to lead interventions locally.

Clinicians are the first key players in the improvement of antibiotic prescribing. To be effective, stewardship programmes should be integrated into existing medical specialities. The role of local non-infection specialist champions in leading best practice is perhaps the strategic cornerstone. Clinicians adhere to locally drawn lines of authority when it comes to prescribing decisions for their patients [26]. This decision is often mainly driven by the experience of seniors rather than guidelines. These cultural rules determining antibiotic prescribing are called 'the prescribing etiquette' [27]. Therefore, an incentive to change behaviours in prescribing may be to acknowledge local hierarchies and include opinion leaders within medical specialities in setting up policies and guidelines in prescribing.

The role of hospital pharmacists in antibiotic stewardship programmes varies across countries and hospitals. Their knowledge and experience in delivering safety and quality improvement initiatives should be used to ensure optimized antimicrobial usage. Pharmacists are in charge of the design and development of decision architectures in prescribing. Using pharmacy resources across specialities can help augment the organizational efforts in optimizing antibiotic usage, with a transverse overview of hospital-wide practices.

Microbiologists constitute the keystone of a good antibiotic stewardship programme. These specialists advise clinicians with a balanced vision on the efficiency and the ecological aspects of antibiotic prescribing. Their reactivity in giving answers and providing diagnosis to clinicians is essential. The drawback is that not all hospitals have onsite microbiology laboratory facilities and lack of access to this essential resource may have an impact on prescribing behaviours [26].

Epidemiologists play a critical role in monitoring data and controlling antibiotic consumption. Their contribution is essential for the purpose of surveillance of antibiotic resistance and consumption.

Neglected key stakeholders

To date, nurses have not been involved in antibiotic stewardship interventions. However, their contribution could improve practice. The role of nurses as organizational knowledge brokers is recognized [28]. They are being increasingly involved in improving quality of care. Highly expert individual nurses acting as antibiotic stewardship consultants can help bring the evidence regarding optimal antibiotic use into the sphere of nursing practice. They may also encourage and spread the wider adoption of increased skills and responsibilities for all nurses.

Social scientists are somewhat neglected participants in antibiotic stewardship programmes. An understanding and application of the social sciences is essential in developing and implementing interventions for behavioural change in antibiotic stewardship. These methods have been widely used in surgery to understand and improve teamwork and patient safety in the operating theatre. Tools such as checklists or team training using simulation have proved their efficacy in preventing complications [29].

Knowledge and the role of education

Influence of knowledge on antibiotic prescribing

A physician's knowledge might influence antibiotic use: a lack of familiarity with or awareness of available evidence or consensus on appropriate antibiotic use might negatively affect prescribing behaviour. Physicians might not know enough about infectious diseases, the potential causative microorganisms, their susceptibility to antibiotic agents, or antibiotic drugs [30]. In teaching hospitals, junior staff (interns and residents) frequently make prescribing decisions even though hospital inpatients are becoming more acutely ill and their cases increasingly complex. The first priority then becomes 'prevention of disaster within the next 24 hours', a goal often thought to be best met by broad-spectrum antibiotics or 'a cacophony of narrow-spectrum agents used in combination'. This approach encourages excessive use of antibiotics [31].

Influence of education

Education, experience, and confidence could be described as factors that influence adherence to infection management pathways. If we add to these the difficulties of diagnosis, many clinicians tend to prefer the route of certainty when prescribing. Interviews with professionals showed that the determinants of the choice of the empirical regimen were that 'everyone feels safe with a broad-spectrum antibiotic; colleagues will not criticize you for this choice', and that, 'we are afraid of missing things, afraid to take risks with our patients, no matter what the guideline recommends' [32]. Diagnostic uncertainty was also described as key driver of drug use and misuse [33]. Fear of being sued for not prescribing an antibiotic, or prescribing the wrong antibiotic, is more common in the USA than in Europe. Prescription decisions seem to be based primarily on instructions passed down through a hierarchical system and subsequently on personal experience

[34]. Formal education, rationale for use, existing guidelines, and concerns about emerging resistance seem to have minor influence [34]. Other investigators have recorded that most clinicians presume that the patient's immediate risk outweighs the long-term disadvantages of the liberal use of antibiotics.

How to educate?

The undergraduate curriculum and internship/foundation year seem optimal stages to build a solid knowledge base for later practice. Conversely, the task of changing the behaviour of trained medical practitioners is very difficult, with multiple barriers [35]. Close collaboration between healthcare providers and academics is needed to link the undergraduate and postgraduate programmes. In hospitals, all the key players described earlier must be involved in the development and implementation of a local educational programme on prudent antibiotic prescribing.

At the postgraduate level, education is an essential element determining antibiotic prescribing behaviour. Persuasive methods of education are usually more popular among clinicians than restrictive measures [30]. Passive education alone (lectures, educational events, leaflets and hand-outs) without the incorporation of active intervention are ineffective. The rapid turnover of junior staff and the difficulty of maintaining a local continuous educational programme are the main reasons for the limited success of in-hospital education. Printed educational materials and educational meetings alone have also had little effect on changing prescribing practices. Face-to-face and one-on-one educational sessions have proved to be a practical, effective, and safe method of reducing excessive use of broad-spectrum antibiotics, but it are costly and labour-intensive [36].

Summary—how to proceed in practice

The above highlights the diverse and complicated social and cultural determinants that influence antibiotic prescribing outcomes in secondary care. The relationship is not a simple pharmacological one that, for example, dictates the course of action in treating diabetes or cancer. Instead, antibiotic prescribing and therapy are beleaguered by many different factors from the social and psychological to the organizational and financial. What is clear is that to preserve the efficacy of this finite class of drugs we need to take action to optimize usage. To do this in the most efficient way involves a better understanding of the cultural and social principles that underpin antibiotic prescribing behaviours among hospital doctors. Interventions to influence prescribing need to be developed within the context in which they are to function. For that, researchers and healthcare professionals need to engage with the local teams and specialities within their organization to ensure that the desired change in behaviour is achieved through mutually agreed goals and targets as part of a clear and deliverable action planning exercise. Being able to assign the right answer to the 'who', 'what', 'where', and 'how' elements of an intervention will ensure that ambiguity is removed, and that, in response to the clarity of expectations, individuals can become more pro-active partners in the intervention.

Currently very few interventions in antibiotic prescribing (which aim to change prescribing behaviours) apply any theory to justify their approach. Knowing the cultural and social context at the local level will enable the use of appropriate behaviour change concepts and approaches to develop interventions that are targeted to specific and local gaps in practice.

The healthcare workforce in hospitals is expanding. In addition to doctors and surgeons, nurses, pharmacists, bench scientists, epidemiologists, and social scientists should be encouraged to be involved in developing safer and more efficacious pathways of patient care. To get the most from this multi-professional team-working concept, healthcare organizations need to invest in postgraduate on-the-job training and education to ensure that their healthcare staff are up to date with evidence-based practice in antibiotic prescribing and infection prevention and control. Policy and guidelines should not be the only repository of information for healthcare professionals.

References

1 Steinke D, Davey P. Association between antibiotic resistance and community prescribing: a critical review of bias and confounding in published studies. *Clin Infect Dis* 2001;33(Suppl. 3):S193–S205.

2 World Health Organization. *The growing threat of antimicrobial resistance: options for action*. 2012. Available at: http://whqlibdoc.who.int/publications/2012/9789241503181_eng.pdf

3 Charani E, Edwards R, Sevdalis N, Alexandrou B, Sibley E, Mullett D, et al. Behavior change strategies to influence antimicrobial prescribing in acute care: a systematic review. *Clin Infect Dis* 2011;53:651–62.

4 Davey P, Peden C, Charani E, Marwick C, Michie S. Time for action-Improving the design and reporting of behaviour change interventions for antimicrobial stewardship in hospitals: early findings from a systematic review. *Int J Antimicrob Agents* 2015;45:203–12.

5 Morris ZS, Clarkson PJ. Does social marketing provide a framework for changing healthcare practice? *Health Policy* 2009;91:135–41.

6 Wise R, Hart T, Cars O, Streulens M, Helmuth R, Huovinen P, et al. Antimicrobial resistance. Is a major threat to public health. *Br Med J* 1998;317:609–10.

7 Hysong SJ, Best RG, Pugh JA. Audit and feedback and clinical practice guideline adherence: making feedback actionable. *Implement Sci* 2006;1:9.

8 Patel SJ, Saiman L, Duchon JM, Evans D, Ferng Y-H, Larson E. Development of an antimicrobial stewardship intervention using a model of actionable feedback. *Interdisexrp Perspect Infect Dis* 2012;2012:150367.

9 Dixon-Woods M, Leslie M, Tarrant C, Bion J. Explaining matching Michigan: an ethnographic study of a patient safety program. *Implement Sci* 2013;8:70.

10 Cars O, Mölstad S, Melander A. Variation in antibiotic use in the European Union. *Lancet* 2001;357:1851–3.

11 Hofstede G. *Culture's consequences: comparing values, behaviors, institutions, and organizations across nations*. Thousand Oaks, CA: Sage Publications; 2001.

12 Kooiker S, van der Wijst L. *Europeans and their medicines*, 2003. Dongen: Social and Cultural Planning Office of the Netherlands.

13 Deschepper R, Vander Stichele R. Differences in use of antibiotics in Europe: the role of cultural aspects. *Pharm Weekbl* 2001;136:794–7.

14 Davey P, Brown E, Charani E, Fenelon L, Gould IM, Holmes A, et al. Interventions to improve antibiotic prescribing practices for hospital inpatients. *Cochrane Database Syst Rev* 2013, (4):CD003543. doi: http://dx.doi.org/10.1002/14651858.CD003543.pub3

15 van Hulst L, Creemers M, Fransen J. How to improve DAS28 use in daily clinical practice?—a pilot study of a nurse-led intervention. *Rheumatology* 2010;49:741–8.

16 Halm EA, Switzer GE, Mittman BS, Walsh MB, Chang CC, Fine MJ. What factors influence physicians' decisions to switch from intravenous to oral antibiotics for community-acquired pneumonia? *J Gen Intern Med* 2001;16:599–605.

17 Majumdar SR, Simpson SH, Marrie TJ. Physician-perceived barriers to adopting a critical pathway for unity-acquired pneumonia. *Jt Comm J Qual Saf* 2004;30:387–95.

18 Shekelle PG, Pronovost PJ, Wachter RM, McDonald KM, Schoelles K, Dy SM, et al. The top patient safety strategies that can be encouraged for adoption now. *Ann Intern Med* 2013;158:365–8.

19 Charani E, Cooke J, Holmes A. Antibiotic stewardship programmes—what's missing? *J Antimicrob Chemother* 2010;65:2275–7.

20 Lorencatto F, West R, Bruguera C, Michie S. Assessing quality of goal setting in smoking cessation behavioural support interventions delivered in practice and associations with quit attempts. Presentation at the UK Society of Behavioural Medicine Annual Conference Oxford 2013.

21 Weinberg M, Fuentes JM, Ruiz AI, Lozano FW, Angel E, Gaitan H, et al. Reducing infections among women undergoing cesarean section in Colombia by means of continuous quality improvement methods. *Arch Intern Med* 2001 22;161:2357–65.

22 Ivers N, Jamtvedt G, Flottorp S, Young JM, Odgaard-Jensen J, French SD, et al. Audit and feedback: effects on professional practice and healthcare outcomes. *Cochrane Database Syst Rev* 2012;(6):CD000259.

23 Dixon-Woods M, Leslie M, Bion J, Tarrant C. What counts? An ethnographic study of infection data reported to a patient safety program. *Milbank Q* 2012;90:548–91.

24 De Vries H, Eggers SM, Bolman C. The role of action planning and plan enactment for smoking cessation. *BMC Public Health* 2013;13:393.

25 Fuller C, Michie S, Savage J, McAteer J, Besser S, Charlett A, et al. The Feedback Intervention Trial (FIT)—improving hand-hygiene compliance in UK healthcare workers: a stepped wedge cluster randomised controlled trial. *PLoS One* 2012;7(10):e41617.

26 Wertheim HFL, Chandna A, Vu PD, Pham CV, Nguyen PDT, Lam YM, et al. Providing impetus, tools, and guidance to strengthen national capacity for antimicrobial stewardship in Viet Nam. *PLoS Med* 2013;10(5):e1001429.

27 Charani E, Castro-Sanchez E, Sevdalis N, Kyratsis Y, Drumright L, Shah N, et al. Understanding the determinants of antimicrobial prescribing within hospitals: the role of 'prescribing etiquette'. *Clin Infect Dis* 2013;57:188–96.

28 Waqa G, Mavoa H, Snowdon W, Moodie M, Schultz J, McCabe M, et al. Knowledge brokering between researchers and policymakers in Fiji to develop policies to reduce obesity: a process evaluation. *Implement Sci* 2013;8:74.

29 Mayer EK, Sevdalis N, Rout S, Caris J, Russ S, Mansell J, et al. Surgical checklist implementation project: the impact of variable WHO checklist compliance on risk-adjusted clinical outcomes after national implementation: a longitudinal study. *Ann Surg* 2016;263:58–63.

30 Pulcini C, Williams F, Molinari N, Davey P, Nathwani D. Junior doctors' knowledge and perceptions of antibiotic resistance and prescribing: a survey in France and Scotland. *Clin Microbiol Infect* 2011;17:80–7.

31 Mattick K, Kelly N, Rees C. A window into the lives of junior doctors: narrative interviews exploring antimicrobial prescribing experiences. *J Antimicrob Chemother* 2014;69:2274–83.

32 Schouten JA, Hulscher MEJL, Natsch S, Grol RPTM, van der Meer JWM. Antibiotic control measures in Dutch secondary care hospitals. *Neth J Med* 2005;63:24–30.

33 Harbarth S, Samore MH. Antimicrobial resistance determinants and future control. *Emerg Infect Dis* 2005;11:794–801.

34 De Souza V, MacFarlane A, Murphy AW, Hanahoe B, Barber A, Cormican M. A qualitative study of factors influencing antimicrobial prescribing by non-consultant hospital doctors. *J Antimicrob Chemother* 2006;58:840–3.

35 Cabana MD, Rand CS, Powe NR, Wu AW, Wilson MH, Abboud PA, et al. Why don't physicians follow clinical practice guidelines? A framework for improvement. *J Am Med Assoc* 1999;282:1458–65.

36 Solomon DH, Van Houten L, Glynn RJ, Baden L, Curtis K, Schrager H, et al. Academic detailing to improve use of broad-spectrum antibiotics at an academic medical center. *Arch Intern Med* 2001;161:1897–902.

Chapter 4

Implementing an antimicrobial stewardship programme

Patrick Doyle

Introduction to antimicrobial stewardship programmes

Antimicrobial stewardship programmes (ASPs) should be at the heart of all antimicrobial initiatives in an institution, be it audit, educational, or 'interdepartmental and interdisciplinary communication and collaboration' pertaining to antimicrobials [1]. Setting up an ASP or expanding it from a small base can be a daunting task. The reasons for this, and the basic principles of antimicrobial stewardship, have been discussed in Chapters 1 and 2 and the necessary interventions on the shop floor will be discussed in Chapter 5. This chapter sets out how to implement an ASP in an individual healthcare setting. Implementing an ASP follows the principles of change management: plan, do, study, act (PDSA) [2].

Know your environment and organization

Before embarking on the development of an ASP, the programme team needs to understand and define their environment and organization.

Information that should be collected includes:

- Patient mix: what patient population does the organization care for, are they primarily surgical or medical, are they long-term care patients, are there large numbers of immune-compromised or elderly patients? These factors will affect where you focus the ASP.

- Antimicrobial consumption: this should be standardized using agreed consumption metrics such as daily defined dose (DDD) (see Chapter 6). Where are the areas of high antimicrobial consumption? Who are the high prescribers? Where are broad-spectrum antimicrobials used?

- Familiarity with local epidemiological patterns and knowledge of infections such as *Clostridium difficile* and antimicrobial resistance rates informs antimicrobial choice and reduces the risk. It is only then that effective targeting, de-escalation, and discontinuation of therapy can be advised, all elements of what Paterson, citing Parrino, describes as the 'back-end approach' to antimicrobial stewardship [3].

- Resources: what resources, both human and funding, are available within the organization to deliver an ASP.

- A gap analysis can be undertaken of existing programmes against potential performance. There are a number of tools available to do this [4,5].

Box 4.1 lists the the most important references to consult when initiating an ASP.

Box 4.1 Practical points

The following resources, all available on the internet, are very useful in implementing an ASP:

◆ 'Antimicrobial stewardship in Australian hospitals' (Australia) [6]

◆ 'Core elements of hospital antibiotic stewardship programs' (CDC, USA) [7]

◆ 'Starting and growing your antimicrobial stewardship program' (Canada) [8]

◆ 'Start smart—then focus' (UK) [5]

◆ 'A hospital pharmacist's guide to antimicrobial stewardship programs' (USA) [9]

Source: data from Public Health England 2015 [5]; Duguid M and Cruickshank M 2015 [6]; Centers for Disease Control and Prevention 2014 [7]; Antimicrobial Stewardship Program 2015 [8]; and American Society of Hospital Pharmacists 2015 [9].

Developing a case for an ASP and gaining support

You must be clear why you are developing an ASP and be able to effectively sell your idea to the institutional stakeholders. Developing a case requires a different emphasis on the core message for different audiences within the organization. The clinical teams are more likely to be responsive to issues of patient safety and antimicrobial resistance. Management are more likely to respond to the financial implications, and this is an important area to consider if you are putting forward a business case to support an ASP.

Patient safety

While patient safety may appear a more ethereal outcome, and therefore difficult to quantify, it is one that every ASP programme needs to have as its focus. The WHO report from the Strategic and Technical Advisory Group on Antimicrobial Resistance (STAG-AMR) makes this abundantly clear [10]. Australian national guidance also states this very unequivocally 'Antibiotic stewardship resides within the healthcare facility's quality improvement and patient safety governance structure' [6]. Owens [11] points out how 'shepherding precious resources' benefits safety and costs, as do George et al. [12] in an intensive therapy unit (ITU) setting.

National campaigns in both Scotland and Wales (the Saving 1000 Lives Campaign) have placed stewardship front and centre as the nucleus of patient safety programmes [13]. Tamma et al. [14] argue that the centrality of patient safety to antimicrobial stewardship is under-emphasized.

In order to work, ASPs must be based on consensus. Commitment is required from management, clinical leadership, and individual healthcare practitioners. Prescribers must feel that they have ownership of programmes and policies [15,16]. Dutch experience has shown that timely and appropriate participation of physicians promotes success, at least with antimicrobial guidance [17].

Financial savings

In times of austerity, interventions to reduce costs will always garner support from healthcare managers saddled with the need to balance budgets. Goff [18] talks about addressing the concerns of those who might oppose an ASP and arbitrating with them by emphasizing the positive outcomes such as improved quality of care, a reduction in drug resistance, and cost savings.

In a university hospital study, Lee et al. [19] showed that implementing the Centers for Disease Control (CDC) antibiotic 'time out' initiative saved money and gave focus to antibiotic targeting [19]. In a study conducted in a Hong Kong hospital in 2008, Ng et al. [20] showed that the human resource costs required to run an ASP could be offset by savings from antibiotic expenditure. Beardsley et al. [21] calculated savings of between USD 900 000 and more than USD 2 000 000 per year with an ASP programme, while Standiford et al. [22] showed that in 7 years of operation an ASP introduced at the University of Maryland Medical Center showed a reduction in antimicrobial expenditure of around USD 3 000 000 in the first 3 years. Despite this, the ASP was terminated, only to be reinstated when cost-effectiveness data became available. Non-cash-releasing benefits flowed from all of these studies but they are harder to quantify.

Requirements for Success

Duguid and Cruickshank [6] in their guide to antimicrobial stewardship in Australian hospitals cite Boaden et al.'s [23] 'factors' for successful improvements of clinical processes and outcomes in healthcare. These are:

1. The need for the participation of a nexus of physicians.
2. The need for individual practitioner feedback.
3. The need for a responsive and supportive organizational culture.
4. The need for appropriate funding and allocation of resources combined with phased, targeted interventions and progress monitoring allowing rapid directional change if needed.
5. The need for an organization's policies to support the efforts and activities of the patient-facing implementers.

Composition of an antimicrobial management team

At its core, antimicrobial stewardship is a multifaceted, multidisciplinary systematic approach to antimicrobial optimization. In Chapter 2 the overall structure of an antimicrobial management team (AMT) was discussed, but a more detailed look is warranted here.

The Infectious Diseases Society of America (IDSA) and Society for Healthcare Epidemiology of America (SHEA) guidelines 2007 [24], reflecting a US setting, emphasized the importance of an infectious diseases (ID) physician and a clinical pharmacist with ID training as essential components of an ASP. Other stakeholders, although important and desirable, were not initially indispensable.

Nathwani [25] emphasized the need for a lead acute hospital doctor and specialist pharmacist together with a medical infection specialist (medical microbiologist and/or ID doctor) as a component of the AMT. He realized that there were few ID physicians in the UK environment and that in this setting medical microbiologists tend to take a leading role.

Clinical pharmacists outnumber microbiology and ID staff and are ideally placed to act as the 'boots on the ground' as they conduct their ward visits interacting with prescribers in what Patterson called the 'trenches' [26,27] and influencing those who actually administer the medicines, i.e. nurses. They are in a unique position to be able to interdict prescribing, often prospectively, by policing the agreed formulary and proposing therapeutic alternatives (the so-called front-end approach) [26].

Charani and Holmes [28] go further, believing that proper engagement in ASPs requires wider involvement, in particular from general pharmacists and nurses. Charani et al. [29], Edwards et al. [30], and Manning [31] all see the forgotten nursing resource as a force multiplier in helping ASPs to develop and succeed, especially in areas where other resources may be threadbare.

Rohde et al. [32] agree with Nathwani that, in the absence of optimal leaders such as ID physicians and ID pharmacists, general 'hospitalists' (internal medicine doctors) and other health professionals can and do make appropriate leaders for ASPs. Rohde et al. argue that enhanced collaboration between hospitalists and ID physicians could fill an unmet need that would allow more institutions to engage in active stewardship programmes. The recommendations from the seminal paper of Dellit et al. [24] that an ASP should be led by an ID physician/ID pharmacist has ironically been seen as a barrier by some establishments to initiating an ASP, especially if they lack those specialist staff.

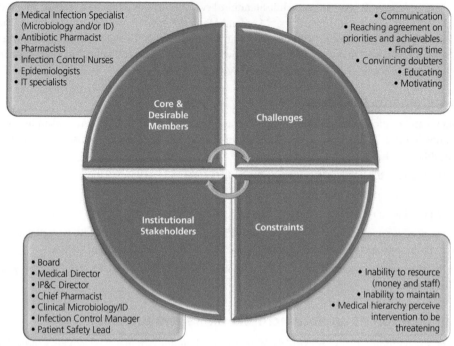

Figure 4.1 Elements and obstacles in implementing an ASP (IP&C, infection prevention and control).

The terms antimicrobial management team and antimicrobial stewardship team (AST) are often used interchangeably, and the exact definition varies from source to source, but a distinction should be drawn between the operational team providing the stewardship on the shop floor and the overall institutional ASP team. However, in many institutions they may comprise the same people (Figure 4.1).

Creating a framework

Allerberger et al. [33] set out a common framework on the structure and organizational requirements to ensure antimicrobial optimization.

Key principles were formulated which remain essential parts of all ASPs:

1. The creation of an organizational framework to lead, endorse, remain accountable for, and specify the scope of action, the direction, the competencies, and activities. The support of hospital management was considered highly desirable.

2. Ensuring there is sufficient capacity in terms of human, material, and technical resources available to proceed.

AMTs should sit at the hub of the governance wheel, as discussed in Chapter 2. Ideally the operational team should have oversight from a group such as an antimicrobial stewardship committee (ASC) which has hospital management and senior clinical representation as well as the members of the AMT (see Figure 4.1).

Communication

Morris et al. [34] state that the AMT should create a vision of their ASP to effectively define its purposes, beliefs, and values, and this can be encapsulated in a vision statement that 'sets the themes and direction for team members' [35]. An example of a vision statement is that from the Mount Sinai Hospital and University Health Network in Toronto, Canada: 'Helping patients receive the right antibiotics when they need them' [35]. It is important that this vision is communicated to all the relevant stakeholders in the institution including senior and middle management, medical, pharmacy, and nursing staff. Methods of communication include newsletters, educational sessions, the internet, and social media (see Chapter 8). The message must be repeated and varied to maintain interest.

Getting started

In 'Antimicrobial stewardship in Australian hospitals', van Gessel and Duguid, citing Boaden et al. [6,23], again describe how one should 'start low and go slow', looking out for the following:

* aim for achievability
* ensure improvement or failure is communicated to participants
* realistic target reconnaissance to drive change
* PDSA cycles to test changes
* know when to enshrine the change.

Changes should be small and introduced sequentially. Each change should be tested *in situ*, using a PDSA cycle to see how it has performed and to allow unforeseen problems to surface [2]. These problems can then be dealt with before proceeding to the next change. It may take several PDSA cycles before full successful implementation is achieved.

Measuring progress

Measurement and feedback of stewardship interventions is essential to the successful implementation of an ASP. These should be both process measures, such as the number of interventions, the number of antimicrobial stewardship rounds completed, and the number of patients reviewed, and outcome measures, such as antimicrobial consumption, resistance rates, and quality of patient care. These are discussed in Chapter 7.

Implementation barriers and how to overcome them

ASPs require patience and determination from the usually limited teams involved in them. One must never discount inspiration and previous experience as drivers for success.

Potential barriers to implementing ASPs include lack of resources in terms of time, funding, or staffing, apathy, ignorance, or a belief that such programmes are too difficult to implement or have little effect on patient flow [36]. Those most willing to engage in antimicrobial stewardship may not have the influence or kudos within the establishment to bring about necessary change management or summon the support to engender the best possibility of success.

Resistance to change is minimized if social aspects are understood, for example perceived attack on prescriber autonomy, and communication is maximized and education strengthened [2,6] (see Chapter 3).

There must be some form of contingency planning should the project run into apathy or opposition or both. In those cases, in order to stay on track, even with a leaner proposal, 'adaptive leadership' [37] will be required. This is where influencing strategies and networking with acquaintances (particularly if strategically placed) can help. The author's own experiences of helping to set up an ASP in the face of some internal friction necessitated the 'stick to one's guns' approach to slowly win over the non-believers. In order to gain executive and senior management support quickly, some achievable gains are required, the so-called 'low hanging fruit' [38]. Initiatives such as switching from intravenous to oral dosing, formulary restriction policies, antibiotic redundancy, and awareness of bioavailability are relatively easy to implement—and more importantly are associated with cash-releasing efficiency savings. Achievements such as this appeal to all 'lean'-thinking healthcare organizations.

Entrenching the programme

Once the initial objectives of the ASP have been met, the strategy must be developed to take the programme forward. Examples include expanding the programme into more challenging areas such as haematology/oncology and antifungal stewardship. Many of these areas are discussed in later chapters. It is vital that the lessons learnt and successes are disseminated to as broad an audience as possible [34].

References

1 File TMJr, Solomkin JS, Cosgrove SE. Strategies for improving antimicrobial use and the role of antimicrobial stewardship programs. *Clin Infect Dis* 2011;**53**(Suppl. 1):S15–S22.

2 Langley G, Moen R, Nolan K, Nolan T, Norman C, Provost L. *The improvement guide: a practical approach to enhancing organizational performance*, 2nd edn, 2009. San Francisco: Jossey-Bass.

3 Paterson DL. Restrictive antibiotic policies are appropriate in intensive care units. *Crit Care Med* 2003;**31**(Suppl. 1):S25–S28.

4 Centers for Disease Control and Prevention. **Antimicrobial management program gap analysis checklist**, 2014. Available at: http://www.cdc.gov/getsmart/healthcare/improve-efforts/resources/pdf/AMP-GapAnalysisChecklist.pdf (accessed 23 March 2015).

5 Public Health England. *Start smart—then focus. Antimicrobial stewardship toolkit for English hospitals*, 2015. Available at: https://www.gov.uk/government/uploads/system/uploads/attachment_data/file/417032/Start_Smart_Then_Focus_FINAL.PDF (accessed March 2015).

6 Duguid M, Cruickshank M. *Antimicrobial stewardship in Australian hospitals*, 2011. Available at: http://www.safetyandquality.gov.au/wp-content/uploads/2011/01/Antimicrobial-stewardship-in-Australian-Hospitals-2011.pdf (accessed April 2015).

7 Centers for Disease Control and Prevention. Core elements of hospital antibiotic stewardship programs, 2014. Available at: http://www.cdc.gov/getsmart/healthcare/implementation/core-elements.html (accessed 23 May 2015).

8 MSH + UHN ASP. Starting and growing your antimicrobial stewardship program, 2015. Available at: http://www.antimicrobialstewardship.com/starting-and-growing-your-antimicrobial-stewardship-program-asp (accessed 17 May 2015).

9 American Society of Hospital Pharmacists. *A hospital pharmacist's guide to antimicrobial stewardship programs*, 2015. Available at: http://www.ashpadvantage.com/docs/stewardship-white-paper.pdf (accessed 25 May 2015).

10 World Health Organization. *Strategic and Technical Advisory Group on Antimicrobial Resistance (STAG-AMR). Report of second meeting 14–16 April 2014*. Available at: http://www.who.int/drugresistance/stag/meeting_summary042014/en/

11 Owens RCJr. Antimicrobial stewardship: application in the intensive care unit. *Infect Dis Clin North Am* 2009;**23**:683–702.

12 George P, Morris AM. Pro/con debate: should antimicrobial stewardship programs be adopted universally in the intensive care unit? *Crit Care* 2010;**14**(1):205.

13 **Infection Management Coalition.** The trinity of infection management: United Kingdom coalition statement, 2014. Available at: http://antibiotic-action.com/wp-content/uploads/2013/09/The-trinity-of-infection-management-final-0913.pdf (accessed 18 May 2015).

14 **Tamma PD, Holmes A, Ashley ED.** Antimicrobial stewardship: another focus for patient safety? *Curr Opin Infect Dis* 2014;**27**:348–55.

15 **Goldmann DA, Weinstein RA, Wenzel RP, Tablan OC, Duma RJ, Gaynes RP, et al.** Strategies to prevent and control the emergence and spread of antimicrobial-resistant microorganisms in hospitals. A challenge to hospital leadership. *J Am Med Assoc* 1996;**275**:234–40.

16 **MacDougall C, Polk RE.** Antimicrobial stewardship programs in health care systems. *Clin Microbiol Rev* 2005;**18**:638–56.

17 **Mol PG, Wieringa JE, Nannanpanday PV, Gans RO, Degener JE, Laseur M, et al.** Improving compliance with hospital antibiotic guidelines: a time-series intervention analysis. *J Antimicrob Chemother* 2005;**55**:550–7.

18 **Goff DA.** Antimicrobial stewardship: bridging the gap between quality care and cost. *Curr Opin Infect Dis* 2011;**24**(Suppl. 1):S11–S20.

19 **Lee TC, Frenette C, Jayaraman D, Green L, Pilote L.** Antibiotic self-stewardship: trainee-led structured antibiotic time-outs to improve antimicrobial use. *Ann Intern Med* 2014;**161**(Suppl. 10):S53–S58.

20 **Ng CK, Wu TC, Chan WM, Leung YS, Li CK, Tsang DN, et al.** Clinical and economic impact of an antibiotics stewardship programme in a regional hospital in Hong Kong. *Qual Saf Health Care* 2008;**17**:387–92.

21 **Beardsley JR, Williamson JC, Johnson JW, Luther VP, Wrenn RH, Ohl CC.** Show me the money: long-term financial impact of an antimicrobial stewardship program. *Infect Control Hosp Epidemiol* 2012;**33**:398–400.

22 **Standiford HC, Chan S, Tripoli M, Weekes E, Forrest GN.** Antimicrobial stewardship at a large tertiary care academic medical center: cost analysis before, during, and after a 7-year program. *Infect Control Hosp Epidemiol* 2012;**33**:338–45.

23 **Boaden R, Harvey G, Moxham C, Proudlove N.** *Quality improvement: theory and practice in healthcare*, 2008. Available at: http://www.nhsiq.nhs.uk/resource-search/publications/quality-improvement-theory-and-practice-in-healthcare.aspx (accessed March 2015).

24 **Dellit TH, Owens RC, McGowan JEJr, Gerding DN, Weinstein RA, Burke JP, et al.** Infectious Diseases Society of America and the Society for Healthcare Epidemiology of America guidelines for developing an institutional program to enhance antimicrobial stewardship. *Clin Infect Dis* 2007;**44**:159–77.

25 **Nathwani D, Scottish Medicines Consortium (SMC) Short Life Working Group, Scottish Executive Health Department Healthcare Associated Infection Task Force.** Antimicrobial prescribing policy and practice in Scotland: recommendations for good antimicrobial practice in acute hospitals. *J Antimicrob Chemother* 2006;**57**:1189–96.

26 **Paterson DL.** The role of antimicrobial management programs in optimizing antibiotic prescribing within hospitals. *Clin Infect Dis* 2006;**42**(Suppl. 2):S90–S95.

27 **Waters CD.** Pharmacist-driven antimicrobial stewardship program in an institution without infectious diseases physician support. *Am J Health-Syst Pharm* 2015;**72**:466–8.

28 **Charani E, Holmes AH.** Antimicrobial stewardship programmes: the need for wider engagement. *BMJ Qual Saf* 2013;**22**:885–7.

29 **Charani E, Castro-Sanchez E, Holmes A.** The role of behavior change in antimicrobial stewardship. *Infect Dis Clin North Am* 2014;**28**:169–75.

30 **Edwards R, Drumright L, Kiernan M, Holmes A.** Covering more territory to fight resistance: considering nurses' role in antimicrobial stewardship. *J Infect Prev* 2011;**12**:6–10.

31 **Manning ML.** The urgent need for nurse practitioners to lead antimicrobial stewardship in ambulatory health care. *J Am Assoc Nurse Pract* 2014;**26**:411–13.

32 **Rohde JM, Jacobsen D, Rosenberg DJ.** Role of the hospitalist in antimicrobial stewardship: a review of work completed and description of a multisite collaborative. *Clin Ther* 2013;35:751–7.

33 **Allerberger F, Gareis R, Jindrak V, Struelens MJ.** Antibiotic stewardship implementation in the EU: the way forward. *Expert Rev Anti Infect Ther* 2009;7:1175–83.

34 **Morris AM, Stewart TE, Shandling M, McIntaggart S, Liles WC.** Establishing an antimicrobial stewardship program. *Healthcare Q* 2010;13(2):64–70.

35 **MSH + UHN ASP.** Starting and growing your antimicrobial stewardship program. Steps 3 and 4: create and communicate the vision, 2015. Available at: http://www.antimicrobialstewardship.com/steps-3-and-4-create-and-communicate-vision (accessed 17 May 2015).

36 **Bal AM, Gould IM.** Antibiotic stewardship: overcoming implementation barriers. *Curr Opin Infect Dis* 2011;24:357–62.

37 **Heifetz RA, Grashow A, Linsky M.** The theory behind the practice. A brief introduction to the adaptive leadership framework. In: *The practice of adaptive leadership: tools and tactics for changing your organization and the world*, 2009, pp. 1–4. Boston, MA: Harvard Business Press.

38 **Goff DA, Bauer KA, Reed EE, Stevenson KB, Taylor JJ, West JE.** Is the 'low-hanging fruit' worth picking for antimicrobial stewardship programs? *Clin Infect Dis* 2012;55:587–92.

Section 2

Components of an antimicrobial stewardship programme

Chapter 5

Managing antimicrobials on the shop floor

Antonia Scobie, Mark Gilchrist, Laura Whitney, and Matthew Laundy

Introduction to managing antimicrobials on the shop floor

The aim of all antimicrobial stewardship programmes is that antimicrobial prescriptions should be safe, rational, and effective and that the unintended consequences of antimicrobial use should be minimized.

There are a number of tools included in national guidelines that can assist healthcare organizations to plan and implement their stewardship strategies [1–4]. The Cochrane Collaboration has also reviewed literature published prior to 2007 [5] and provides a summary of the evidence to support different stewardship strategies.

The actual methods used to manage antimicrobials on the shop floor vary widely between institutions and countries, and depend on the healthcare setting, its priorities, and the resources allocated to stewardship. The availability of services with sufficient capacity to take on stewardship activities, such as diagnostics, onsite microbiology laboratories, medical infection specialists, and clinical pharmacy services, will have a significant impact on which strategies are chosen and implemented. Particular consideration should be given to the accessibility of such services when planning interventions, as centres with 24-hour microbiology and pharmacy services will be able to employ different tactics from those with time-restricted or offsite services.

In addition to a formal antimicrobial management team (AMT) structure (discussed in Chapter 2), it may be valuable to create a team that can practically monitor and manage antimicrobial use.

The shop floor team should be a multidisciplinary team reflecting those skills in the formal AMT. The team needs a leader who is qualified, motivated, and assertive on both a clinical and a management level. Ideally a senior medical specialist should lead the reviews, as antimicrobial recommendations are likely to be more conservative and have lower acceptance rates when made by unsupervised trainees [6].

Implementation of any new stewardship strategy to manage antimicrobials on the shop floor should always be carefully planned, with efforts made to solicit support within the organization (from clinicians and management) and predict, identify, and manage any unintended consequences.

Reducing inappropriate antimicrobial use

Reducing inappropriate antimicrobial usage is the key to stewardship. Several methods of reducing inappropriate antimicrobial use have been suggested, including preventing the initiation of or stopping unnecessary treatment, restricting durations to the shortest effective course, and reducing the use of broad-spectrum antimicrobials.

Preventing the initiation of antimicrobials

The withholding of antimicrobials can be encouraged by using local or national guidelines to highlight conditions that do not require antimicrobial treatment. This strategy has been widely employed for outpatients and surgical prophylaxis, but may also be utilized for inpatients. Providing clear case definitions and encouraging the use of diagnostic tests can assist prescribers in differentiating between infections where antimicrobial therapy is indicated and those where it is not [1].

One method of preventing the initiation of antibiotics is the suppression of antimicrobial susceptibility results on specimens not thought to be clinically relevant (see Chapter 10).

There has been increasing interest in the potential for biomarkers to assist the decision to start antimicrobials. This is discussed further in Chapter 17.

Reducing the duration of treatment

This can be achieved in several ways: creating guidelines that advocate the shortest appropriate course is an easy first step in this process. There is good evidence that shorter courses of antibiotics are as effective as prolonged courses for respiratory tract infections [7–10], uncomplicated urinary tract infections [11], and surgical prophylaxis [12]. Interventions that limit durations can have a significant impact because prescriptions for these infections make up a large proportion of antimicrobial use [13].

Automatic stop orders, which cease antibiotic therapy after a defined period of time, and separate antibiotic prescription charts, which allow only a limited treatment duration, have also been shown to be effective in reducing antibiotic consumption and increasing documented reviews [14–16]. However, such interventions should be implemented carefully in strictly defined patient groups to prevent morbidity associated with early cessation of therapy.

The encouragement of clinical review and cessation of antimicrobials when infection is ruled out or cured are more challenging aspects, but can be achieved with antimicrobial stewardship rounds (covered later in this chapter) or an infectious diseases review [17]. Improved documentation of the indication for, and proposed duration of, therapy has been advocated to assist the review process [1], as has the use of reminder stickers in medical notes [18].

Reducing unnecessary broad-spectrum treatment: formulary restriction

Restrictive strategies have been shown to outperform persuasive strategies in the stewardship setting [5]. Formulary restriction and pre-authorization is one such restrictive strategy that has had success in the clinical setting. It has been introduced in a variety of ways in hospitals (Table 5.1). It is also necessary to consider how compliance with the restrictive policy will be monitored and how non-compliance will be sanctioned.

Such restrictive programmes have been shown to reduce consumption of restricted agents by up to 95%, with corresponding reductions in healthcare-associated infections such as *Clostridium difficile*, vancomycin-resistant enterococci, and extended spectrum β-lactamase-producing coliforms [19–21].

It is important to support restriction by removing restricted agents from clinical guidelines and ward stocks wherever possible. Clearly, this must be balanced by allowing restricted agents to be used when they are the optimum therapy and ensuring availability to allow prompt treatment

Table 5.1 Formulary restriction strategies

	Explanation	Advantages	Disadvantages
Types of restriction			
1. Pre-authorization	The 'restricted antibiotic' cannot be initiated without approval by infection specialists or pharmacists	Likely to have most impact on usage	Can delay treatment Difficult to maintain out of hours as requires 24/7 microbiology/ID/pharmacy cover and there may be difficulties contacting prescribers out of hours
2. Authorization for continued use	Anyone may prescribe a restricted agent; however, usage beyond a specified time-point requires review and approval	Avoids potential for delaying antibiotics in severe infections and associated risks	Can be difficult to stop/de-escalate antibiotics once initiated if patient improves Easier to circumnavigate restrictions
Restrictive methodologies			
1. Pharmacy managed	Notes review to check for approval prior to supply	No new charts/software, etc. required for implementation	Time-consuming for pharmacy Difficult to manage out of hours and without ward-based pharmacy services if using paper medical notes Potential for delays whilst prescriber contacted if not clear in notes
2. Authorization codes	Microbiology give out a code, which must be documented on the drug chart before supply	Less open to abuse than the above method Can be used without ward-based pharmacy services	Codes can be 'made up' Can be difficult to double-check codes—may require a shared database between pharmacy and microbiology
Methods of supporting restriction			
1. Prospective audit	Through ward-based audit or post-discharge review of medical notes	Most robust method	Time-consuming Requires good documentation of approval process in notes
2. Feedback on unapproved use only	Requires identification from pharmacists/ward based staff with mechanisms for reporting and sanctions	Easy to implement	Ad hoc nature is likely to limit success as all misuse may not be reported or followed up
3. Stewardship rounds	The multidisciplinary stewardship team reviews use of restricted antimicrobials and feeds back on their use	Allows clinical review of cases Feedback to prescribers in person and on actual cases of inappropriate use may be more successful as an educational strategy Can cross-check that approval of the drug was appropriate	Time-consuming Requires expertise, preferably MDT Will not capture all inappropriate use May be difficult to identify patients for review

(continued)

Table 5.1 Continued

	Explanation	Advantages	Disadvantages
4. Cross-checking prescriptions/ issues from pharmacy with approvals	Provision of a list of restricted antibiotics dispensed from pharmacy or identified from electronic prescribing systems for confirmation by those approving the drugs	Circumnavigates problems of poor documentation in notes Can prompt reviews, either by microbiology/ID or as part of MDT ward rounds	Requires pharmacy or prescribing software Unlikely to be an exhaustive list (antibiotics may be used from stock or borrowed from another patient) Data accuracy issues (i.e. antibiotics booked out to the wrong patient may be included in the list, lists may not be timely) May be complex if more than one team is involved in the approval process

ID, infectious disease; MDT, multidisciplinary team.

when prescribed appropriately. Strategies to manage this include having exemptions for certain indications, for example cephalosporins for meningitis, without the need for approval, and ensuring either a rapid supply from a 24-hour pharmacy service or maintaining accessible stock in areas likely to be initiating treatment. It is also imperative to adequately communicate the introduction of any new restrictive process to prescribers and nursing and pharmacy staff.

Potential pitfalls of restrictive strategies that must be considered prior to introduction include:

◆ delayed treatment for patients, with potentially increased morbidity and mortality

◆ increased consumption of alternative agents, with different adverse effects on both individual patients and the ecology of the hospital

◆ increased pressure on microbiology and pharmacy departments to manage the process

◆ additional prescribing complexity by requiring prescribers to navigate the approval system

◆ increased nursing time due to travelling to collect antibiotics

◆ changes in empiric guidelines may lead to more complex administration processes.

Persuasive strategies include audit and feedback (A&F). A&F is a commonly used approach for changing the behaviour of healthcare professionals. A systematic review examining the effectiveness of different stewardship interventions (89 studies) found that interventions aimed at increasing effective prescribing for pneumonia were associated with reduced mortality risk while interventions aimed at reducing excessive prescribing were not [5]. Many of the intervention studies published to date lack fundamental details on how the interventions were delivered; a recent systematic review found that only 13.8% of intervention studies specifically included feedback of data to participants [22].

Using evidence-based guidelines and clinical pathways to standardize practice

A widely accepted and adopted component of stewardship programmes is the development of evidenced-based guidelines/policies to aid prudent prescribing [1,3,4,23]. In addition, the development of clinical pathways can instil a standard approach to reduce variations in treatment. Such pathways can also play a role in patient safety and can help to reduce potential antimicrobial resistance and the development of healthcare-associated infections.

Guidelines and clinical pathways should be developed with both the infection team and the end user in mind and should be jointly agreed and championed, with support from senior hospital management and approval from local stewardship committees or equivalent. Such guidelines and pathways should be subject to regular review taking into account new evidence, changes in local resistance patterns, or clinical incidents resulting in a breach in care.

Whilst the antimicrobials within empirical and specialist guidelines may differ the core principles should not. Typically these should contain elements around the following:

- *general prescribing principles* related to the need for an antimicrobial, considering a non-infective inflammatory diagnosis
- *reviewing microbiology samples* both past and present to help direct therapy by either broadening or narrowing spectra and switching or stopping agents
- *documenting a clear antimicrobial plan*—communicating why the antimicrobial is indicated together with an intended duration (consideration should be given to forming an antimicrobial plan in the medical records, which should be reviewed daily)
- *sepsis* and how life-threatening infection should be effectively managed
- *allergies*—offering alternatives for patients with an allergy (most commonly penicillin)
- *de-escalation strategies*—such as intravenous to oral switch programmes or, where possible, outpatient parenteral antimicrobial therapy (OPAT) (the criteria for both strategies should be clearly defined)
- *minimizing the use of broad-spectrum antimicrobials* to prevent healthcare-associated infections, e.g. *C. difficile*
- *therapeutic drug monitoring* advice for antibiotics such as aminoglycosides and glycopeptides
- *surgical prophylaxis*—promoting the use of a single dose where possible
- *contact information* for medical and pharmacy teams to discuss cases with their local infection or stewardship team.

Intravenous to oral switch programmes

Switching to an oral agent minimizes the need for an intravenous device, which may be associated with catheter-related bloodstream infections. Moreover, an early switch reduces treatment complexity and can (for soft tissue and respiratory infections) lead to savings in drug acquisition costs and nursing time without impacting on clinical care [24–26].

For a switch to be effective and safe, the oral agent should have good bioavailability and be known to be effective against the identified or presumed pathogen. It should be able to reach appropriate concentrations at the site of infection and should not be used where there is a lack of evidence for the indication. Furthermore, the patient should be responding to their initial therapy without any malabsorption concerns [24,25]. Box 5.1 lists the criteria for intravenous to oral switch.

Audit and feedback

Audit

This involves post-prescription review, and comparing the use, choice, and planned duration against a standard of practice—either locally or nationally accepted guidelines. Traditionally the review takes place 48–72 hours post-prescription so that culture, radiology, and other results are

---

Box 5.1 When to switch to oral therapy

Criteria for intravenous to oral switch:

◆ clinical improvement has been observed

◆ there is not a condition-specific contraindication to oral therapy

◆ oral fluids are tolerated

◆ temperature has been within normal limits for at least 24 hours

◆ no unexplained tachycardia and heart rate < 100 b.p.m. for at least 12 hours

◆ white cell count between 4 and 12×10^9/L and C-reactive protein returning to normal range

◆ no on-going or potential problems with absorption

◆ a suitable oral antimicrobial is available which will penetrate to the site of the infection

Exclusions to intravenous to oral switch:

◆ patients with compromised oral absorption

◆ continuing decompensated sepsis

◆ endocarditis

Relative contra-indications to switch or indications for a delayed switch:

◆ meningitis/encephalitis/brain abscess

◆ osteomyelitis/septic arthritis/bone or joint infections/infected implants/prostheses/graft tissue

◆ complex skin and soft tissue infections

◆ deep abscess

◆ bloodstream infections

Source: data from Desai M et al., 'A new approach to treatment of resistant gram-positive infections: potential impact of targeted IV to oral switch on length of stay', *BMC Infectious Diseases*, 6:94, Copyright © 2006 Desai et al.; licensee BioMed Central Ltd.

---

available to guide treatment decisions. The optimal timing of feedback is debatable given a recent study showing reduced all-cause and infection-related mortality at 30 days when review occurred within 48 hours of antibiotic prescription [27]. Review may not always be possible within this time frame; therefore it may be more realistic to conduct ward rounds at regular defined intervals (e.g. three times a week).

The list of patients requiring review can be generated from pharmacy dispensary records of restricted antimicrobials, from pre-authorization patient lists, clinician, nurse, or ward pharmacist request, review of charts to identify all patients on antimicrobials, reporting tools linked to electronic health records, and clinical decision support systems (see Chapter 8).

Feedback

The overall effects of A&F on the practice of health professionals are modest; however, feedback is most effective when it is provided, both verbally and in written format, from a supervisor or colleague, more than once, when the baseline performance is low and with well-defined targets and an action plan [28]. Feedback is also more effective when one is hoping to decrease rather than increase behaviours and when it is delivered soon after the event—so the healthcare provider

Box 5.2 What should be fed back about antimicrobial prescribing

The following points should be fed back at an antimicrobial stewardship round:

◆ appropriateness of the decision to initiate antimicrobial therapy

◆ appropriateness of the choice of agent and adherence to local guidelines

◆ discontinuation of antibiotics

◆ intravenous to oral switch

◆ de-escalation from broad-spectrum to narrow-spectrum agent

◆ dose optimization

◆ therapeutic monitoring

◆ actions to reduce the risk of hospital acquired infection, e.g. prompt removal of intravenous and urinary catheters

can actually recall the details of the case; larger effects are also seen when trying to modify simple behaviours, such as prescribing, compared with complex practices, such as test ordering [28].

In order for feedback to be 'actionable', i.e. effective at changing the behaviour of a healthcare care professional, it needs to be:

◆ timely—delivered a minimum of monthly

◆ individualized—delivered to the actual prescriber

◆ non-punitive—educational and constructive to the recipient

◆ customisable—to enable the recipient to understand the data that are fed back to them [29].

Additional influential factors include specific suggestions for improvement or the provision of the correct solution [30]. Rates of acceptance of feedback are reported to be lower when the recommendations involve discontinuation rather than modification of therapy [31].

The difficulty in providing feedback to some units, for example intensive care, is that while junior team members complete the prescriptions, the prescribing decisions are often made at a senior level. Juniors may be uncomfortable about questioning decisions even if they are aware that the antimicrobial does not adhere to local policy. The hierarchical structure of many clinical units presents difficulties in providing individualized feedback, as the prescriber may not feel accountable for that prescribing decision. In such situations it may be more useful to provide feedback to the senior members of the team as well rather than just to the individual prescriber (Box 5.2).

Advice on relevant infection control practices such as isolation and precaution

A&F can be done as a one- or two-stage process. In a one-stage process, the antimicrobial stewardship team (AST) performs the review as part of a designated stewardship round. In a two-stage process there may be an initial review by an infectious disease (ID) pharmacist and any complex cases or cases that meet defined criteria will be identified for further review by the AMT.

Prior to implementation of A&F, there needs to be appropriate consultation with the recipients of the feedback to increase the likelihood of endorsement. At first there may be reluctance by clinical teams to adopt such recommendations; however, with regular interaction over time, perceptions and behaviour eventually change. In some cases, prescribing behaviour may shift to the other end of the spectrum where almost all antimicrobial prescribing decisions are deferred to infection specialists, and additional resources may need to be allocated to accommodate this behaviour shift.

Performing audit and feedback: the 'antimicrobial stewardship round'

This is often the most utilized approach. For the round to be most effective, the prescriber should be present on the round so cases can be discussed, reviewed, and relevant verbal feedback provided immediately. In situations where prescribers are not available, the round may involve a review of a patient's medical records and results with feedback written in the medical notes or communicated directly to the prescriber via telephone, e-mail, or text.

The effectiveness of the round is often dependent on the personality and communication style of the 'steward'. An assertive steward is likely to bring about more changes in antimicrobial prescribing; however, if they are too confrontational this may result in unsafe practices such as premature discontinuation of antibiotics prior to scheduled review dates so juniors don't have to present cases. On the other hand, if a steward is meek or too supportive there is likely to be no change in prescribing practice.

The main advantage of performing a clinical round is that it enables real-time feedback to the prescriber and prompt modification of antimicrobial therapy. In the majority of settings acceptance of feedback recommendations remains voluntary, which allows prescribers to retain a degree of autonomy in initiating empiric treatment. The round can also be used as a teaching tool for junior prescribers regarding certain aspects of diagnosis and management of patients with infections.

The main disadvantage of the stewardship round is that it is labour-intensive and expensive when performed on a regular basis. Further funding may be needed to provide the additional personnel (such as an antimicrobial pharmacist) to meet these requirements. Other issues include: potential deterioration in inter-departmental relations when clinicians are made to justify their management decisions to other healthcare professionals; the primary team may be uncomfortable taking advice when the patient may not have been fully assessed by the AMT; and teams may be reluctant to stop or de-escalate treatment if their patient has improved on current therapy for fear of 'rocking the boat'. The voluntary nature of advice acceptance means that one is unlikely to see immediate effects in antimicrobial usage unless the rounds are accompanied by other strategies such as formulary restriction or pre-authorization.

There are a variety of approaches to conducting a stewardship round; these can be categorized into regular and targeted rounds.

Regular scheduled ward rounds in units with high antimicrobial usage

Units such as intensive care, haematology, oncology, and acute medicine are obvious areas to review. This may involve reviewing all patients receiving antimicrobials in the unit or, if there are time constraints, patients who have recently been commenced on antibiotics (e.g. those admitted on a medical take). The number of regular rounds can be adjusted according to need and resources, for example one to three times a week. During the implementation phase, areas with the highest antimicrobial usage can be targeted first and then the frequency of rounds can be increased as appropriate.

An essential component of effective stewardship rounds is endorsement from senior colleagues of the relevant specialities. This may be difficult to obtain at first; a potential solution is to select a representative from that speciality to act as a stewardship lead who can be approached with specific issues. The rounds need to occur regularly as prescribing practices may quickly revert to the baseline if there are periods with no stewardship presence. Likewise, if they are not frequent enough, correct practice may only occur prior to the round rather than throughout the week.

The advantage of a regular round is that it enables trust to develop in the stewardship team, thus rates of acceptance of recommendations may increase over time. It also enables review of cases requiring more complex antimicrobial input due to drug–disease factors or drug–drug interactions. One of the disadvantages of a dedicated stewardship ward round is that it often only involves junior clinicians, thus the opportunity to target senior colleagues (who may be driving most of the prescription decisions) will be missed.

Targeted rounds

Antimicrobial-directed round Depending on resources, patients receiving any broad-spectrum antimicrobial or just those receiving selected 'restricted' antimicrobials (e.g. quinolones, cephalosporins, or carbapenems) can be selected for review. Cases can be identified through pharmacy records or pre-authorization databases. Once the review is complete, feedback can be verbally communicated to the team or documented in the patient's records.

Results-targeted round This may involve reviewing patients following isolation of pathogens or multidrug-resistant organisms from significant sites, for example the bloodstream or other sterile sites that will likely require prolonged antimicrobial therapy.

The advantage of these strategies is that they are not dependent on the schedules of other clinical teams; the rounds can be performed when convenient for the AST and can be focused solely on stewardship. On the other hand, as the clinical team are unlikely be present at the time of review, the process of gathering information from a patient's chart is labour-intensive and potentially inefficient. Additionally, whilst there is less potential for confrontation, the lack of direct communication may result in recommendations being missed or ignored by the clinical team.

Targeting areas with high rates of healthcare-associated infections This can include concentrating antimicrobial review to units with either: (1) high rates of colonization (with or without subsequent infection) with drug-resistant organisms (e.g. meticillin-resistant *Staphylococcus aureus*, vancomycin-resistant enterococci, or carbapenem-resistant *Enterobacteriaceae*) or (2) hospital-acquired *C. difficile* infection. An advantage of this strategy is that infection control practices can be simultaneously reviewed and fed back.

Outpatient parenteral antimicrobial therapy

OPAT is a treatment option for patients who are medically fit for hospital discharge but require prolonged parenteral antimicrobials, enabling shortened or avoided hospital stays. There are adult and paediatric guidelines/good practice recommendations that illustrate the key themes for running OPAT services [32–34].

Reviewing patients for their suitability for OPAT provides an ideal opportunity to review antimicrobial use for de-escalation to narrower-spectrum antimicrobials, intravenous to oral switch, or even antimicrobial cessation. OPAT should practice stewardship principles including the optimization and reporting of outcomes, healthcare-associated infections, and re-admission rates [35]. Conversely, there is a risk that using OPAT services may actually increase the use of particular broad-spectrum agents—those possessing pharmacokinetic properties enabling once daily dosing—over more suitable narrow-spectrum antimicrobials.

Using OPAT as a stewardship opportunity is a more collaborative approach as the clinical team are already requesting an antimicrobial review when referring patients. The drawback is that it is too sporadic—cases where patients in whom OPAT is not appropriate will not get referred and will therefore be missed. Additionally, many of the patients who are referred may already have received prolonged courses of inappropriate therapy by the time they are referred.

References

1 **Public Health England**. *Start smart—then focus. Antimicrobial stewardship toolkit for English hospitals*, 2015. Available at: https://www.gov.uk/government/uploads/system/uploads/attachment_data/file/417032/Start_Smart_Then_Focus_FINAL.PDF (accessed March 2015).

2 **Centers for Disease Control and Prevention**. Core elements of hospital antibiotic stewardship programs. 2014. Available at: http://www.cdc.gov/getsmart/healthcare/implementation/core-elements.html (accessed May 2015).

3 **Duguid M, Cruickshank M.** *Antimicrobial stewardship in Australian hospitals*. 2011. Available at: http://www.safetyandquality.gov.au/wp-content/uploads/2011/01/Antimicrobial-stewardship-in-Australian-Hospitals-2011.pdf (accessed April 2015).

4 **Dellit TH, Owens RC, McGowan JEJr, Gerding DN, Weinstein RA, Burke JP, et al.** Infectious Diseases Society of America and the Society for Healthcare Epidemiology of America guidelines for developing an institutional program to enhance antimicrobial stewardship. *Clin Infect Dis* 2007;44:159–77.

5 **Davey P, Brown E, Charani E, Fenelon L, Gould IM, Holmes A, et al.** Interventions to improve antibiotic prescribing practices for hospital inpatients. *Cochrane Database Syst Rev* 2013;(4):CD003543.

6 **Yeo CL, Wu JE, Chung GW, Chan DS, Fisher D, Hsu LY.** Specialist trainees on rotation cannot replace dedicated consultant clinicians for antimicrobial stewardship of specialty disciplines. *Antimicrob Resist Infect Control* 2012;1:36.

7 **el Moussaoui R, de Borgie CA, van den Broek P, Hustinx WN, Bresser P, van den Berk GE, et al.** Effectiveness of discontinuing antibiotic treatment after three days versus eight days in mild to moderate-severe community acquired pneumonia: randomised, double blind study. *Br Med J* 2006;332:1355.

8 **Choudhury G, Mandal P, Singanayagam A, Akram AR, Chalmers JD, Hill AT.** Seven-day antibiotic courses have similar efficacy to prolonged courses in severe community-acquired pneumonia—a propensity-adjusted analysis. *Clin Microbiol Infect* 2011;17:1852–8.

9 **Chastre J, Wolff M, Fagon JY, Chevret S, Thomas F, Wermert D, et al.** Comparison of 8 vs 15 days of antibiotic therapy for ventilator-associated pneumonia in adults: a randomized trial. *J Am Med Assoc* 2003;290:2588–98.

10 **Micek ST, Ward S, Fraser VJ, Kollef MH.** A randomized controlled trial of an antibiotic discontinuation policy for clinically suspected ventilator-associated pneumonia. *Chest* 2004;125:1791–9.

11 **Lutters M, Vogt N.** Antibiotic duration for treating uncomplicated, symptomatic lower urinary tract infections in elderly women. *Cochrane Database Syst Rev* 2002;(3):CD001535.

12 **Scottish Intercollegiate Guidelines Network**. *Antibiotic prophylaxis in surgery*. Guideline **104**. 2014. Available at: http://sign.ac.uk/guidelines/fulltext/104/index.html (accessed 24 March 2015).

13 **ESAC-3: Hospital Care Subproject Group**. *Report on point prevalence survey of antimicrobial prescribing in European hospitals, 2009*. 2009. Available at: http://ecdc.europa.eu/en/activities/surveillance/ESAC-Net/publications/Documents/report_survey_antimicrobial_prescriptions_eu_hospitals_2009.pdf (accessed April 2015).

14 **Ashiru-Oredope D, Richards M, Giles J, Smith M, Teare L.** Does an antimicrobial section on a drug chart influence prescribing? *Clin Pharmacist* 2011;3:222.

15 **Durbin WA Jr, Lapidas B, Goldmann DA.** Improved antibiotic usage following introduction of a novel prescription system. *J Am Med Assoc* 1981;246:1796–800.

16 **Echols RM, Kowalsky SF.** The use of an antibiotic order form for antibiotic utilization review: influence on physicians' prescribing patterns. *J Infect Dis* 1984;150:803–7.

17 **Lesprit P, de Pontfarcy A, Esposito-Farese M, Ferrand H, Mainardi JL, Lafaurie M, et al.** Postprescription review improves in-hospital antibiotic use: a multicenter randomized controlled trial. *Clin Microbiol Infect* 2015;21:180.e1–180.e7.

18 Pulcini C, Defres S, Aggarwal I, Nathwani D, Davey P. Design of a 'day 3 bundle' to improve the reassessment of inpatient empirical antibiotic prescriptions. *J Antimicrob Chemother* 2008;**61**:1384–8.

19 Dancer SJ, Kirkpatrick P, Corcoran DS, Christison F, Farmer D, Robertson C. Approaching zero: temporal effects of a restrictive antibiotic policy on hospital-acquired *Clostridium difficile*, extended-spectrum beta-lactamase-producing coliforms and meticillin-resistant *Staphylococcus aureus*. *Int J Antimicrob Agents* 2013;**41**:137–42.

20 Aldeyab MA, Kearney MP, Scott MG, Aldiab MA, Alahmadi YM, Darwish Elhajji FW, et al. An evaluation of the impact of antibiotic stewardship on reducing the use of high-risk antibiotics and its effect on the incidence of *Clostridium difficile* infection in hospital settings. *J Antimicrob Chemother* 2012;**67**:2988–96.

21 Quale J, Landman D, Saurina G, Atwood E, DiTore V, Patel K. Manipulation of a hospital antimicrobial formulary to control an outbreak of vancomycin-resistant enterococci. *Clin Infect Dis* 1996;**23**:1020–5.

22 Davey P, Peden C, Charani E, Marwick C, Michie S. Time for action—improving the design and reporting of behaviour change interventions for antimicrobial stewardship in hospitals: early findings from a systematic review. *Int J Antimicrob Agents* 2015;**45**:203–12.

23 NHS Institute for Improvement and Innovation. Quality and improvement tools: protocol based care. 2008. Available at: http://www.institute.nhs.uk/quality_and_service_improvement_tools/quality_and_service_improvement_tools/protocol_based_care.html (accessed April 2015).

24 Dryden M, Saeed K, Townsend R, Winnard C, Bourne S, Parker N, et al. Antibiotic stewardship and early discharge from hospital: impact of a structured approach to antimicrobial management. *J Antimicrob Chemother* 2012;**67**:2289–96.

25 Desai M, Franklin BD, Holmes AH, Trust S, Richards M, Jacklin A, et al. A new approach to treatment of resistant gram-positive infections: potential impact of targeted IV to oral switch on length of stay. *BMC Infect Dis* 2006;**6**:94.

26 Seaton RA, Bell E, Gourlay Y, Semple L. Nurse-led management of uncomplicated cellulitis in the community: evaluation of a protocol incorporating intravenous ceftriaxone. *J Antimicrob Chemother* 2005;**55**:764–7.

27 Liew YX, Lee W, Tay D, Tang SS, Chua NG, Zhou Y, et al. Prospective audit and feedback in antimicrobial stewardship: is there value in early reviewing within 48 h of antibiotic prescription? *Int J Antimicrob Agents* 2015;**45**:168–73.

28 Ivers N, Jamtvedt G, Flottorp S, Young JM, Odgaard-Jensen J, French SD, et al. Audit and feedback: effects on professional practice and healthcare outcomes. *Cochrane Database Syst Rev* 2012;(6):CD000259.

29 Hysong SJ, Best RG, Pugh JA. Audit and feedback and clinical practice guideline adherence: making feedback actionable. *Implement Sci* 2006;**1**:9.

30 Hysong SJ. Meta-analysis: audit and feedback features impact effectiveness on care quality. *Med Care* 2009;**47**:356–63.

31 Cosgrove SE, Seo SK, Bolon MK, Sepkowitz KA, Climo MW, Diekema DJ, et al. Evaluation of postprescription review and feedback as a method of promoting rational antimicrobial use: a multicenter intervention. *Infect Control Hosp Epidemiol* 2012;**33**:374–80.

32 Chapman AL, Seaton RA, Cooper MA, Hedderwick S, Goodall V, Reed C, et al. Good practice recommendations for outpatient parenteral antimicrobial therapy (OPAT) in adults in the UK: a consensus statement. *J Antimicrob Chemother* 2012;**67**:1053–62.

33 Patel S, Abrahamson E, Goldring S, Green H, Wickens H, Laundy M. Good practice recommendations for paediatric outpatient parenteral antibiotic therapy (p-OPAT) in the UK: a consensus statement. *J Antimicrob Chemother* 2015;**70**:360–73.

34 Tice AD, Rehm SJ, Dalovisio JR, Bradley JS, Martinelli LP, Graham DR, et al. Practice guidelines for outpatient parenteral antimicrobial therapy. IDSA guidelines. *Clin Infect Dis* 2004;**38**:1651–72.

35 Gilchrist M, Seaton RA. Outpatient parenteral antimicrobial therapy and antimicrobial stewardship: challenges and checklists. *J Antimicrob Chemother* 2015;**70**:965–70.

Chapter 6

Measuring antibiotic consumption and outcomes

Hayley Wickens

Introduction to measuring antibiotic consumption and outcomes

In order to assess the effects of an antimicrobial stewardship programme, it is necessary to monitor antimicrobial usage, processes, and outcomes.

Consumption, issues, or sales?

It is important to differentiate between antimicrobial issue data and consumption data. Issues are measured in terms of prescriptions or volumes of product issued to patients, or in the hospital setting to wards, and are at best a proxy for consumption. It may become possible with the advent of individualized single-dose issuing systems to track accurately the amounts of a drug taken by each patient, in the hospital setting at least. Directly observed therapy has been used for many years for treatment of tuberculosis; however, this is not the norm for other antimicrobials, and it is not unknown for patients to hoard unused medication in the community setting. When looking at national or health system data, it is therefore worth considering how these data were generated—are they reimbursement data (e.g. from prescriptions issued) or even sales data (which may also include stock sitting on shelves unissued)?

DDDS, ADQS, DIDS, and STAR-PUs

Inevitably, the literature on antimicrobial usage is littered with acronyms. The World Health Organization lists a 'defined daily dose' (DDD) for the vast majority of medicines available worldwide, and antimicrobials are no exception [1]. These DDDs represent a typical daily dose of each drug for an adult of average weight, and can be used as a numerator when comparing usage of antimicrobials between centres. The major disadvantage of using DDDs to compare usage between settings is that they do not take account of, for example, paediatric usage or units with a high proportion of patients with renal impairment, who will receive a reduced dosage. DDDs may also vary from the doses commonly given in particular countries, and therefore other measures are sometimes used. For instance, in England, average daily quantities (ADQs) are sometimes, but not always, used (see Table 6.1); these are more commonly seen in primary care data analysis than in secondary care, and were calculated for that setting. Average daily doses of these agents may sometimes be higher in hospital usage than in primary care (Table 6.1), highlighting the need to ideally also monitor the number and length of courses, rather than total use as a sole measure.

Days of therapy (DOT) is a measure more commonly used in the USA than the UK, and represents the number of days for which a patient has received the specified antimicrobial. This has

Table 6.1 Defined daily doses (DDD), average daily quantities (ADQ), and some typical hospital total daily doses for antimicrobials (consult product literature before prescribing) [1,2]

Antimicrobial	DDD	ADQ	Typical UK hospital adult daily dose
Amoxicillin (oral)	1 g	750 mg	1.5 g
Azithromycin (oral)	300 mg	500 mg	500 mg
Ciprofloxacin (oral)	1 g	750 mg	1–1.5 g
Ciprofloxacin (IV)	500 mg	–	800 mg
Co-amoxiclav (oral)	1 g as amoxicillin component	3 × 325 mg tablets or 3 × 625 mg tablets	1.5 g expressed as amoxicillin component
Co-amoxiclav (IV)	3 g as amoxicillin component	–	3 g expressed as amoxicillin component
Flucloxacillin (oral)	2 g	1 g	2–4 g (unlicensed)
Metronidazole (oral)	2 g	–	1.2 g
Vancomycin (oral)	2 g	500 mg	0.5–1 g
Vancomycin (IV)	2 g	2 g	2–4 g (unlicensed, depends on serum levels)

IV, intravenous.

Source: data from World Health Organization Collaborating Centre for Drug Statistics Methodology, *ATC/DDD Index 2015*, Copyright © WHO 2015, available from www.whocc.no/atc_ddd_index/; and Health and Social Care Information Centre, *ADQ values 2012/13*, Copyright © 2012, The Health and Social Care Information Centre, Prescribing and Primary Care Services. All rights reserved. Available from: www.hscic.gov.uk/media/9376/Average-daily-quantity-ADQ-values-2012-13/pdf/adqs_2012_13.pdf

the advantage of eliminating variation due to paediatric or renal dosage, or local variation from international DDD values. It is very labour-intensive to quantify DOTs in secondary care in the absence of electronic prescribing systems; however, the number of prescriptions (available from UK primary care data) or packs can act as a proxy for the number of patients treated.

DDDs and ADQs are usually expressed in terms of activity, with the denominator varying by setting. Therefore in secondary care usage will be often expressed as DDDs per 1000 occupied bed days, or 1000 admissions, whilst in studies of primary care DDDs per 1000 inhabitants per day (a measure known as DIDs), or per standardized patient, may be used. Two standardized patient denominator units used in primary care in the UK are STAR-PUs (specific therapeutic group age–sex weightings related prescribing units) and ASTRO-PUs (age, sex and temporary resident originated prescribing unit).

Measuring antimicrobial usage across the UK and Europe

Since the transfer of responsibility for health to the UK devolved administrations, the ways in which antimicrobial data are collated and reported for primary and secondary care have evolved differently in each of the four countries. However, all four are working in response to the UK Department of Health 5-year antimicrobial resistance strategy (2013–18) [3].

Initiatives in the four countries include the following:

♦ NHS National Services Scotland maintains a central register of all prescriptions dispensed in the community (the Prescribing Information System for Scotland, PRISMS) and the Hospital

Medicines Utilisation Database (HMUD), allowing interrogation of prescribing and financial data across both databases. Health Protection Scotland and the Information Services Division of NHS Scotland provide an Antimicrobial Management Integrated Database for Scotland (AMIDS), which provides combined information on antimicrobial prescribing and resistance, in support of improvements in antimicrobial stewardship.

◆ The Welsh Antimicrobial Resistance Programme Surveillance Unit (WARP-SU) collates and reports antimicrobial issue data from hospitals, focusing on inpatient usage, with primary care prescription data obtained from the Prescribing Services Unit of NHS Wales Shared Service Partnership. Point prevalence survey results, along with antimicrobial resistance rates per health board, and per hospital, are published alongside antimicrobial usage data.

◆ The Northern Ireland COMPASS system provides data on primary care antibiotic prescribing at practice, locality, and regional level, as does the national prescribing database. A national antimicrobial resistance dataset is being developed. The Strategy for Tackling Antimicrobial Resistance 2012–17 (STAR) document highlighted the potential for electronic prescribing in hospitals to support integration of prescribing and resistance data.

◆ The first report of ESPAUR (English Surveillance Programme on Antimicrobial Usage and Resistance) was published in 2014, and collated, for the first time, antimicrobial usage and resistance data from both primary and secondary care in England. Further developments are under way to provide an interactive drug usage and resistance database and expand the drug–organism combination lists included in surveillance.

The UK has participated in the European Surveillance of Antimicrobial Consumption (ESAC) project since its inception in 2001 at the University of Antwerp, Belgium. The project transferred to the European Centre for Disease Prevention and Control (ECDC) in 2011 as ESAC-Net; until 2014, collation and submission of primary care usage data from the four UK administrations was organized by the British Society for Antimicrobial Chemotherapy. ESAC-Net collates primary and secondary care antimicrobial usage data from 30 European Union (EU)/European Economic Area countries; related projects hosted by ECDC are HAI-Net (healthcare-associated infection surveillance), HALT-2 (healthcare-associated infection and antimicrobial use in long-term care facilities), and EARS-Net (antimicrobial resistance surveillance).

Other EU countries have local networks for surveillance of antimicrobial consumption and associated resistance data, for example BAPCOC (the Belgian Antibiotic Policy Coordination Committee) and STRAMA (the Swedish Strategic Programme for the Rational Use of Antimicrobial Agents).

The Transatlantic Taskforce on Antimicrobial Resistance (TATFAR), hosted by the US Centers for Disease Control, was established in 2009 to promote cooperation in the promotion of appropriate antibiotic use and development of new agents. It has recommended harmonization of definitions and terminology around antimicrobial usage surveillance (e.g. DDDs and DOTs), prevalence methodology, and resistance surveillance in order to improve transatlantic communication and data sharing worldwide.

Gaps in UK prescribing data

There are currently several gaps in UK antimicrobial prescribing datasets. Private prescriptions are not included in the primary care antibiotic data as the prescription itself is generally retained by the dispensing pharmacy and is therefore not passed to a central service for reimbursement. Similarly, antimicrobial issues in private hospitals are not always included in central government datasets, though these data may be available from commercial organizations (e.g. IMS Health, Danbury, CT, USA).

Data from NHS dental prescribing are available from the same sources as NHS general practice/primary care prescribing; however, as a large proportion of dental services in the UK are delivered on a private basis, prescribing data in this sector are largely limited to commercial sales data.

Surveillance of veterinary use of antimicrobials in the UK and Europe

Measurement of veterinary usage of antimicrobials in the UK is an area subject to development. Currently there is no central collation of veterinary antimicrobial usage; the UK-Veterinary Antibiotic Resistance and Sales Surveillance (UK-VARSS) report gives sales data obtained from manufacturers by the Veterinary Medicines Directorate. Usage is reported in tonnage, with a population correction unit applied to correct for the number, and relative masses, of animals treated. Antimicrobial resistance data are compiled from diagnostic samples and other studies. Twenty-six countries, including the UK, participate in the European Surveillance of Veterinary Antibiotic Consumption (ESVAC) project hosted by the European Medicines Agency. As part of the UK Department of Health 'One Health' initiative, there is an intention to bring human and veterinary antimicrobial usage and resistance data together over the coming years in order to provide a better understanding of the interaction between these fields.

Process and outcome measures in antimicrobial usage

Antimicrobial stewardship is often measured in terms of process indicators, such as correct documentation of indication, correct antimicrobial choice with regard to local guidelines, or administration of the appropriate antibiotic within an hour of a sepsis diagnosis. However, outcome measures are often more difficult to obtain, as these tend to require prospective surveillance of, for instance, clinical or microbiological resolution of infection, 28-day mortality, or readmission for infection-related diagnosis after discharge from hospital. Outside clinical trials, these data may not always be formally collated; improvements in clinical coding and information systems may facilitate this in the future.

Most hospitals in the England conduct point prevalence surveys of antimicrobial use at yearly or more frequent intervals [4]; such studies are based on infection control methodology, and involve all antimicrobial prescriptions in the hospital (or nursing home) setting being reviewed on a single day with regards to dose, documented indication, and guideline compliance. Other epidemiological data may also be collected (e.g. the presence of a urinary or vascular catheter) depending on the needs of the organization. Typically, point prevalence data are collected by clinical pharmacists in the UK on their daily ward visit, but in other countries infection specialist doctors or nurses may collect the data. Robust design of paper, or web-based, data collection forms is key to ensuring a uniform dataset, eliminating ambiguity by specifying in advance, for example, whether to include stat doses, topical agents, or half days of therapy. The most useful data item from such surveys that cannot be generated from raw drug usage data is the prevalence of antimicrobial prescriptions, i.e. the proportion of inpatients receiving an antimicrobial at any one time; longitudinal usage data for antimicrobials is more appropriately generated from dispensing record systems. Prevalence surveys and quality indicators as a tool to improve stewardship will be discussed in more detail elsewhere in this book. The importance and utility of electronic prescribing in measuring antibiotic consumption is self-evident and is discussed in Chapter 8.

References

1 **World Health Organization Collaborating Centre for Drug Statistics Methodology.** ATC/DDD Index 2016. Available at: http://www.whocc.no/atc_ddd_index/

2 **Health and Social Care Information Centre.** ADQ values 2012/13. Available at: http://www.hscic.gov.uk/media/9376/Average-daily-quantity-ADQ-values-2012-13/pdf/adqs_2012_13.pdf

3 **Department of Health and Department for Environment, Food and Rural Affairs.** *UK five year antimicrobial resistance strategy 2013 to 2018*. 2013. Available at: https://www.gov.uk/government/uploads/system/uploads/attachment_data/file/244058/20130902_UK_5_year_AMR_strategy.pdf

4 **Wickens HJ, Farrell S, Ashiru-Oredope DA, Jacklin A, Holmes A** (ASG-ARHAI). The increasing role of pharmacists in antimicrobial stewardship in English hospitals. *J Antimicrob Chemother* 2013; 68:2675–81.

Chapter 7

Measuring and feeding back stewardship

Jacqueline Sneddon and William Malcolm

Introduction to measuring and feeding back stewardship

Measurement is an essential element of any antimicrobial stewardship programme as it enables organizations and clinicians to plan, prioritize, and evaluate the success of their interventions. When planning a stewardship intervention a means of measuring its impact should always be considered. This applies to interventions such as development and implementation of a new guideline, a quality initiative to optimize prescribing, or the launch of a new educational resource to support healthcare staff. The concept of measuring to improve understanding was known as early as the nineteenth century; Lord Kelvin is famously quoted as saying 'if you cannot measure it you cannot improve it'. Measurement has been used for centuries in research but more recently it has become a cornerstone of benchmarking and scrutiny within healthcare. It is also utilized through various means to improve quality and reduce the failure rate in manufacturing industries, and these approaches have become widely used in healthcare. Data capture is a key factor in designing measurement of stewardship interventions. Electronic systems can capture data to provide quantitative information for monitoring longitudinal trends but for many healthcare interventions manual collection of data through clinical audit may be required to support improvement in practice. Electronic data linkage is highlighted within the UK 5-year antimicrobial resistance strategy (2013–18) [1] to provide a true assessment of the intended and unintended impact of stewardship interventions on patient care. Specific measures, ratios, or indicators may also be used to monitor changes over time, between geographical areas, and before and after interventions.

Quality improvement methodology

The use of quality improvement methodology within healthcare has expanded rapidly over the past 10 years, supported by organizations such as the Institute for Healthcare Improvement (IHI) [2] in the USA and The Health Foundation [3] in the UK. Much of the experience and the tools used in quality improvement originated in the manufacturing and aviation industries, which have radically improved safety during the past 25 years.

Data suggesting that one in ten admissions to hospital results in an adverse event are one of the key drivers for improving patient safety in healthcare in the UK [4]. These data provide the impetus to improve practice, reduce errors, and understand near misses. The financial implications of errors, such as costs of litigation and increased length of stay and reputational risks, must also be considered. Interventions involving invasive medical devices and compliance with local policies for both infection control and antimicrobial prescribing have been a focus for quality improvement [5,6]. The primary drivers for improvement are: the 'will' to change, 'ideas' to make processes

---

Box 7.1 Types of measures—with examples related to management of sepsis

- *Outcome measures*: How is the system performing? What is the result? (For example, are patients diagnosed with sepsis receiving a first dose of antibiotic within 1 hour?)
- *Process measures*: Are the parts/steps in the system performing as planned? (For example, are all clinical staff aware of the local sepsis policy and able to access it at the point of care?)
- *Balancing measures*: Looking at a system from different directions/dimensions. What happened to the system as we improved the outcome and process measures? (For example, unanticipated consequences such as outcomes for patients with diagnoses other than sepsis, increased use of broad-spectrum antibiotics)

---

and outcomes better, and the capacity/capability (theories, tools, and techniques) to enable the 'execution' of the ideas. There are several quality improvement methodologies used in healthcare, for example the Model for Improvement, LEAN, and Six Sigma, but all have similar components.

The Model for Improvement provides a simple yet powerful tool for accelerating improvement based on three fundamental questions [7]:

'What are we trying to achieve?' [A clear aim—what, how much, by when?]

'How will we know that change is an improvement?' [Measuring processes and outcomes]

'What changes can we make that will result in an improvement?' [What do we want to test? What can we learn as we go along?]

Improvement is about gathering just enough data, constantly changing what we are doing depending on our small tests of change and using statistical process control tools such as run charts to measure improvement over time. Three types of measure may be used, as shown in Box 7.1.

Structure and process indicators for stewardship

Antimicrobial stewardship is a fairly new concept, and measures of its effectiveness have begun to be developed during the past few years. Several groups in Europe have published structural indicators for hospital stewardship programmes [8–10] and the top 10 validated ones are shown in Box 7.2.

Auditing the quality of prescribing

In the absence of electronic prescribing in hospitals point prevalence surveys (PPS) are used to audit the quality of antimicrobial prescribing. PPS have been used at European [11] and national levels [12] to map trends over time in relation to quality measures such as the percentage of patients receiving an antibiotic, the percentage of intravenous antibiotics, and percentage compliance with local antibiotic policy and to identify local and national priorities for improvement [13].

These high-level data may be useful for feedback within national organizations to inform policy, while results from local surveys can be fed back to managers and clinicians. Audit tools from these PPS can also be utilized to undertake bespoke audits focusing on specific wards or specific antibiotics to support improvement activity.

Antimicrobial prescribing indicators are explicitly defined measureable items of antibiotic use giving a possible indication of the level of quality. The Scottish Antimicrobial Prescribing Group

Box 7.2 Top 10 validated indicators for antimicrobial stewardship in European hospitals

1. Formal mandate for hospital multidisciplinary antimicrobial management team (AMT)

2. AMT member is a member of the drug and therapeutics committee

3. Bedside expert consultant advice regarding antibiotics available on request the same day

4. Regular ward rounds by members of AMT performed at least weekly

5. Clinical audit of prescribers' compliance with local clinical guidelines by the AMT

6. Antibiotic formulary/list updated biannually

7. Local clinical practice guidelines for microbiologically documented therapy updated biannually

8. Local clinical practice guidelines for empirical therapy updated biannually

9. Local clinical practice guidelines for surgical prophylaxis available

10. Prescriber education by personalized interactive methods (e.g. daily ward rounds, face to face training sessions)

Source: data from Buyle F et al., 'Development and validation of potential structure indicators for evaluation antimicrobial stewardship programmes in European hospitals', *European Journal of Clinical Microbiology and Infectious Diseases*, Volume 32, Issue 9, pp. 1161–70, Copyright © 2013 Springer-Verlag Berlin Heidelberg.

has developed national and hospital prescribing quality indicators [14] to support a government target for reduction of *Clostridium difficile* infection; example data are shown in Figure 7.1.

Indicators for hospital stewardship are included in the 'Start Smart then Focus' [6] campaign, and the UK Department of Health has recently proposed prescribing indicators with targets for NHS England. The recent progress report of the Transatlantic Taskforce on Antimicrobial Resistance [15] calls for a global approach to the development of indicators for stewardship as one of its key recommendations.

Indicators to measure the quality of healthcare in community settings are being increasingly used by clinicians and policy makers. A set of 12 quality indicators were developed and validated by the European Surveillance of Antimicrobial Consumption (ESAC) programme [16] and are shown in Box 7.3.

The most useful indicator relating to selection pressure for antimicrobial resistance is consumption of antibacterials for systemic use [Anatomical Therapeutic Chemical (ATC) Classification System code J01]. Other indicators considered in isolation are less useful due to interdependences. In Scotland a national prescribing indicator with a target was introduced in 2013 using a 'best in class' approach to drive improvement [17] and a similar indicator is planned in England.

Antibiotic-specific prescribing indicators may be less relevant for clinicians than for policy makers, therefore the ESAC have also developed a set of disease-specific quality indicators for antibiotic prescribing in primary care [18] (see Box 7.4).

Feedback of data

For all types of audit, regular and timely feedback is essential to drive improvements in practice. Sharing prescribing data with front-line clinicians in real time is the most effective way to allow them to reflect on their practice and encourage them to change their prescribing behaviours.

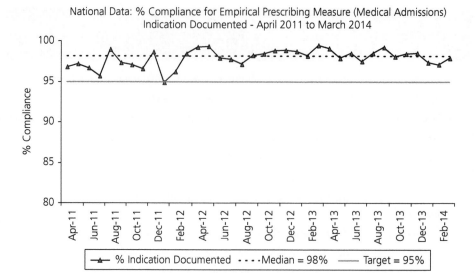

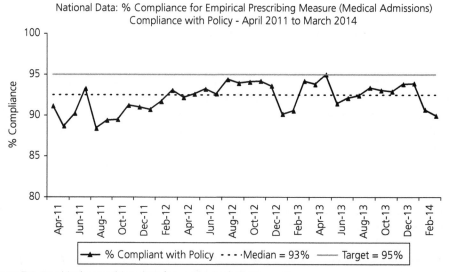

Figure 7.1 Empirical prescribing data for medical admissions units.

Source: data from Institute for Healthcare Improvement extranet website, www.ihi.org.

Comparison with peers and identification of prescribers who are outliers are useful techniques for changing behaviour. Ideally, clinical teams (medical and nursing staff) should collect audit data to give ownership and support improvements in practice. Many methods can be used for feeding back data depending on the audience and whether the data are being used for scrutiny, for example targets, or for quality improvement. Published reports, run charts, and benchmarking tables are examples of feedback outputs (see Box 7.5).

Box 7.3 ESAC-validated primary care quality indicators

- Consumption of antibacterials for systemic use (ATC J01) expressed in defined daily doses per 1000 inhabitants per day (DID)
- Consumption of penicillins (ATC J01 C) expressed as DID
- Consumption of cephalosporins (ATC J01 D) expressed as DID
- Consumption of macrolides, lincosamides, and streptogramins (ATC J01 F) expressed as DID
- Consumption of quinolones (ATC J01 M) expressed as DID
- Consumption of beta-lactamase-sensitive penicillins (ATC J01 CE) expressed as a percentage of total consumption for systemic use (ATC J01)
- Consumption of combination of penicillins including beta-lactamase inhibitors (ATC J01 CR) expressed as a percentage of total consumption for systemic use (ATC J01)
- Consumption of third and fourth generation cephalosporins [ATC J01 (DD+DE)] expressed as a percentage of total consumption for systemic use (ATC J01)
- Consumption of fluoroquinolones (ATC J01 MA) as a percentage of total consumption for systemic use (ATC J01)
- Ratio of the consumption of broad-spectrum {ATC J01 [CR+DC+DD+(F−FA01)]} to the consumption of narrow-spectrum penicillins, cephalosporins, and macrolides [ATC J01 (CE+DB+FA01)]
- Seasonal variation of total antibiotic consumption (ATC J01)
- Seasonal variation of quinolone consumption (ATC J01 M)

Adapted by permission from BMJ Publishing Group Limited: *BMJ Quality and Safety*, Coenen S et al., 'European Surveillance of Antimicrobial Consumption (ESAC): quality indicators for outpatient antibiotic use in Europe', Volume 16, Issue 6, pp. 440–445, Copyright © 2007 BMJ Publishing Group Ltd and The Health Foundation.

Box 7.4 Evidence

- Development and validation of potential structure indicators for evaluation of antimicrobial stewardship programmes in European hospitals (*Eur J Clin Microbiol Infect Dis* 2013;32:1161–70)
- European Surveillance of Antimicrobial Consumption (ESAC): quality indicators for outpatient antibiotic use in Europe (*Qual Saf Health Care* 2007;16:440–5)
- *Start smart—then focus. Antimicrobial stewardship toolkit for English Hospitals.* Public Health England, March 2015 (https://www.gov.uk/government/uploads/system/uploads/attachment_data/file/215308/dh_131181.pdf)

Box 7.5 Practical points

- Make measurement count. Consider who collects data, sample size, frequency, and feedback methods
- Use validated indicators for benchmarking and comparison between hospitals
- Use locally agreed measures for clinical audit

Conclusion

Measurement has become an established part of modern healthcare systems but there is a danger that front-line staff can be swamped by data collection, taking them away from patient care. To ensure that data collection is reliable and sustainable it should be integrated into the daily routine rather than being an extra task. It is also important to ensure that results are visible and fed back to those who collected the information so that staff remain motivated and can be proud of their achievements. Within the field of antimicrobial stewardship, metrics for monitoring structure, process, and outcomes are still evolving. However, there are many examples of good practice that can be followed to provide assurance about the effectiveness of local stewardship programmes.

References

1 **Department of Health and Department for Environment, Food and Rural Affairs.** *UK five year antimicrobial resistance strategy 2013 to 2018.* 2013. Available at: https://www.gov.uk/government/uploads/system/uploads/attachment_data/file/244058/20130902_UK_5_year_AMR_strategy.pdf

2 **Institute for Healthcare Improvement.** URL: http://www.ihi.org/about/Pages/default.aspx

3 **The Health Foundation.** URL: http://www.health.org.uk/

4 **Vincent C, Neale G, Woloshynowych M.** Adverse events in British hospitals: preliminary retrospective record review. *Br Med J* 2001;**322**:517–19.

5 **The Scottish Patient Safety Programme.** URL: http://www.scottishpatientsafetyprogramme.scot.nhs.uk/

6 **Public Health England.** *Start smart—then focus. Antimicrobial stewardship toolkit for English Hospitals.* 2015. Available at: https://www.gov.uk/government/uploads/system/uploads/attachment_data/file/215308/dh_131181.pdf

7 **Institute for Healthcare Improvement.** *How to improve* [The Model for Improvement]. Available at: http://www.ihi.org/resources/Pages/HowtoImprove/default.aspx

8 **Van Gastel E, Costers M, Peetermans WE, Struelens MJ;** Hospital Medicine Working Group of the Belgian Antibiotic Policy Coordination Committee. Nationwide implementation of antibiotic management teams in Belgian hospitals: a self-reporting survey. *J Antimicrob Chemother* 2010;**65**:576–80.

9 **Thern J, de With K, Strauss R, Steib-Bauert M, Weber N, Kern WV.** Selection of hospital antimicrobial prescribing quality indicators: a consensus among German antibiotic stewardship (ABS) networks. *Infection* 2014;**42**:351–62.

10 **Buyle FM, Metz-Gercek S, Mechtler R, Kern WV, Robays H, Vogelaers D,** et al. Development and validation of potential structure indicators for evaluation antimicrobial stewardship programmes in European hospitals. *Eur J Clin Microbiol Infect Dis* 2013;**32**:1161–70.

11 **European Surveillance of Antimicrobial Consumption.** *Report on point prevalence survey of antimicrobial prescribing in European hospitals.* 2009. Available at: http://ecdc.europa.eu/en/activities/surveillance/ESAC-Net/publications/Documents/report_survey_antimicrobial_prescriptions_eu_hospitals_2009.pdf

12 **Health Protection Scotland.** *Scottish national point prevalence survey of healthcare associated infection and antimicrobial prescribing 2011.* 2012. Available at: http://www.documents.hps.scot.nhs.uk/hai/sshaip/prevalence/report-2012-04.pdf

13 **Malcolm W, Nathwani D, Davey P, Cromwell T, Patton A, Reilly J,** et al. From intermittent antibiotic point prevalence surveys to quality improvement: experience in Scottish hospitals *Antimicrob Resist Infect Control* 2013;**2**(1):3.

14 **The Scottish Government.** A revised framework for national surveillance of healthcare associated infection and the introduction of a new health efficiency and access to treatment (heat) target for *Clostridium difficile* associated disease (CDAD) for NHS Scotland. Chief Executive Letter **11**. 2009. Available at: http://www.sehd.scot.nhs.uk/mels/CEL2009_11.pdf

15 **Centers for Disease Control and Prevention**. Transatlantic Taskforce on Antimicrobial Resistance (TATFAR). *TATFAR Progress report 2014*. 2014. Available at: http://www.cdc.gov/drugresistance/tatfar/report.html

16 **Coenen S, Ferech M, Haaijer-Ruskamp FM, Butler CC, Vander Stichele RH, Verheij TJ, et al.** European Surveillance of Antimicrobial Consumption (ESAC): quality indicators for outpatient antibiotic use in Europe. *Qual Saf Health Care* 2007;**16**:440–5.

17 **Scottish Antimicrobial Prescribing Group**. *Primary care prescribing indicators. Annual report 2013–14*, p. 3. 2014. Available at: https://isdscotland.scot.nhs.uk/Health-Topics/Prescribing-and-Medicines/Publications/2014-10-14/2014-10-14-SAPG-Primary-Care-PI-2013-14-Report.pdf

18 **Adriaenssens N, Coenen S, Tonkin-Crine S, Verheij TJ, Little P, Goossens H;** on behalf of the ESAC Project Group. European Surveillance of Antimicrobial Consumption (ESAC): disease-specific quality indicators for outpatient antibiotic prescribing. *BMJ Qual Saf* 2011;**20**:764–72.

Chapter 8

Information technology in antimicrobial stewardship

Matthew Laundy

Introduction to information technology in antimicrobial stewardship

The information technology (IT) revolution has totally changed the way we function in society. Yet sometimes it appears that this revolution has bypassed healthcare, partially due to its inherently conservative nature and partially to justifiable concerns about patient safety and privacy. Many healthcare facilities are still totally or partially reliant on paper-based patient records that are little different from those used 50 years ago.

This is changing. Initiatives such as the Health Information Technology for Economic and Clinical Health (HITECH) Act in the USA [1] and the National Program for IT (NPfIT) in the UK have moved forward the agenda on IT in healthcare. The HITECH approach uses financial incentives to individual practitioners and organizations providing Medicare and Medicaid to adopt electronic health records (EHRs), the so-called meaningful use initiative. The NPfIT took a more top-down approach to implementation within the UK National Health Service (NHS).

The roll-out of electronic records and prescribing provides many opportunities for antimicrobial stewardship (AMS). Figure 8.1 illustrates the sources and flow of information in the healthcare setting relevant to AMS. The use of information technology in AMS is presented in Box 8.1.

Electronic health records

An EHR is a longitudinal electronic record of patient health information generated by one or more encounters in any care delivery setting. Included in this information are patient demographics, progress notes, problems, medications, vital signs, past medical history, immunizations, laboratory data, and radiology reports [2]. The terms electronic patient record (EPR) and electronic medical record (EMR) are often used interchangeably, although there are subtle but important differences. We will use the term EHR as it is all-encompassing.

There are a number of EHR systems available, mostly originating from the USA. Cerner Corporation (Kansas City, MO, USA) and Epic Systems Corporation (Verona, WI, USA) are major providers in the UK and US markets.

For AMS, electronic prescribing of medication (ePrescribing) is the core functionality of an EHR. Beyond this, EHRs in themselves have until recently had little functionality relating to AMS specifically, although this is changing. Cerner Corporation is currently trialling a module for AMS.

The functionality that exists depends on the vendor but often includes:

◆ order sets
◆ compulsory indication entering

- hard stop or review dates
- dose checking
- restricted antimicrobial alerts
- allergy alerts
- links to best practice guidelines
- intravenous to oral algorithms
- documentation of antimicrobial stewardship programme (ASP) interventions.

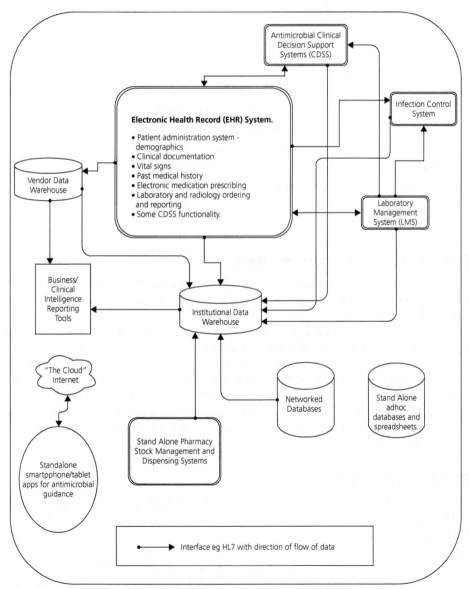

Figure 8.1 Sources and flow of information in the healthcare setting relevant to antimicrobial stewardship.

Box 8.1 Uses of information technology in antimicrobial stewardship

- Alerts to the AMS team of patients prescribed antimicrobials, to support intervention and feedback
- Identification of patients receiving prolonged-antimicrobial treatment
- Identification of infectious syndromes for intervention
- Prescriber decision support including evidence-based antimicrobial guidelines, allergies, important drug interactions, and best practice alerts
- Supporting formulary restriction and pre-authorization
- Capture of indication for antimicrobial use
- Measuring and analysis of antimicrobial consumption at institution, unit, and prescriber levels
- Identifying organism/antimicrobial mismatch, and modifying antimicrobial therapy
- Identifying changes in resistance patterns to guide empiric guideline development
- Documentation of stewardship team intervention
- Gap analysis
- Measurement of ASP interventions
- Quantification of savings by an ASP

Clinical decision support systems

Clinical decision support is a process for enhancing health-related decisions and actions with pertinent, organized clinical knowledge and patient information, to improve health and healthcare delivery [3].

At the simplest level a clinical decision support system (CDSS) in AMS can be access to online guidelines or a smartphone app. However, CDSSs in AMS often refer to specialist, usually commercially produced, systems. Commercial examples include Antibiotic Assistant (Hospira, Lake Forest, IL, USA) and ABXAlert (ICNet, Stroud, UK). These systems are connected to existing clinical systems such as EHRs, laboratory management systems (LMSs), and infection control (IC) systems, as illustrated in Figure 8.1. CDSSs may be a component part of IC software. AMS CDSSs provide some or all of the functions described in Box 8.1 and there is good evidence to support their use (see Box 8.2).

Mobile applications

The ubiquitous smartphone or tablet computer provides an ideal opportunity to guide the prescribing and management of antimicrobials. Commercially available apps such as Sanford Guide (Antimicrobial Inc., Sperryville, VA, USA) and Johns Hopkins ABX (Unbound Medicine, Charlottesville, VA, USA) guides are well known. They have a US bias and do not always reflect local practice. Apps relevant to local antibiotic guidelines can be developed to reflect practice and resistance patterns. Many organizations have developed their own successful in-house antimicrobial apps: one study showed that 100% of junior doctors had downloaded the relevant app

Box 8.2 The evidence for clinical decision support systems in antimicrobial stewardship

- Correct antibiotic [9,10]
- Reduction in antibiotic usage [11–14]
- Reduction in broad-spectrum antibiotic use [15]
- Shorter length of stay [9,11]
- Reduction in adverse events [11,12]
- Decreased mortality [12]
- Increase in pharmacy interventions [11]
- Reduction in time spent on AMS activities by AMT team [11]
- Decreased costs [9,11,13]

Source data from Andreassen PM et al. 2006 [9]; Thursky KA et al. 2006 [10]; Evans RS et al. 1998 [11]; Pestotnik S et al. 1996 [12]; Calloway S et al. 2013 [13]; Schulz L et al. 2013 [14]; and Litvin CB et al. 2013 [15].

by 12 months, the app was accessed 10 times more frequently than the web version, and 71% of clinicians felt that their antibiotic knowledge had improved [4]. In-house development can be hampered by a lack of in-house expertise, but more importantly the loss of expertise rendering the app unsupported. One approach taken by the MicroGuide app (Horizon SP, Leeds, UK) is to provide a framework within which individual organizations can modify content and structure themselves while the technical and hosting aspects are maintained by the developers (see Figure 8.2). Analytical information on who accesses what, when, and where is provided to the organization by the developer to help guide further development.

Barriers to implementation of information technology in antimicrobial stewardship

The cost of IT systems is high, both in their implementation and maintenance, and it is a cost that management is often reluctant to bear. There is often a lack of institutional support, with clinical IT and analysis being seen as less important than financial reporting.

A major barrier is the lack of IT and analytical skills within organizations. IT skills can often be transitory with projects being left unsupported once skilled individuals leave.

Leadership is often lacking both clinically and within IT departments. There is often a lack of clinical buy-in and poor management of change, with clinical teams having little input into decision making.

In many healthcare organizations data are often stored in individual databases or spreadsheets that are inaccessible to all but the users—'data silos'. This leads to duplicated data with inefficiency and inconsistency.

Data security and legislation are important factors to consider. Organizational requirements on the governance of information and legislative regulations dictate what data can be stored and where. Examples of this legislation are the Data Protection Act in the UK and the many federal and state laws in the USA.

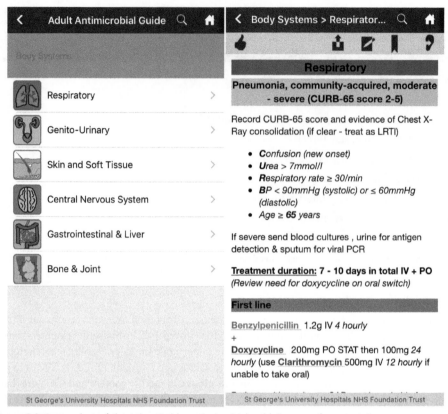

Figure 8.2 Screenshot of the MicroGuide antimicrobial guideline app for smartphones.

Reproduced courtesy of Horizon Strategic Partners Limited.

Social media

Social media applications such as Twitter (San Francisco, CA, USA), Facebook (Menlo Park, CA, USA), and YouTube (Google, Mountainview, CA, USA) have become integral to twenty-first-century life.

Where should one use social media for AMS? One relevant group is medical staff in training—a group most likely to initiate antimicrobials but also one of the most difficult to engage with. They have a high turnover rate, restrictive work hours, and limited time. However, they are also the most likely to have embraced social media and to be users of mobile devices. This provides the AMS team with an opportunity to provide education regarding antimicrobial use. The effectiveness of this approach has not been reported in AMS but its success is well recognized in other areas. Examples of use would include dissemination of information, quizzes, online chats, and re-Tweeting of important research, journal articles, and national and international campaigns.

There are some important points to consider when developing a social media campaign in AMS [5,6]:

- keep it active—if the social media are barely updated, people will not return
- keep it interesting

- ◆ ensure access for all—many organizations block social media
- ◆ ensure activity alignment—all social media should have a similar message
- ◆ integrate the social media campaign with traditional media
- ◆ maintain patient confidentiality
- ◆ avoid specific advice to patients
- ◆ avoid spreading erroneous or biased information.

Online antimicrobial stewardship resources and education

The ability to disseminate information and teach subjects to a vast audience over the internet independent of geography has changed the way we provide education.

The web has a large number of AMS resources, too numerous and ephemeral to list. One recent example is the European Society of Clinical Microbiology and Infectious Diseases (ESCMID) Study Group for Antibiotic Policy Policies (ESGAP) Antimicrobial Stewardship Virtual Learning Community, an open-access web-based resource to provide information and tools to foster AMS [7].

Apart from traditional university courses available online there has been the development of massive open online courses (MOOCs). These are online open-access courses with unlimited enrolment. They can involve online video lectures, notes, and slide presentations. Participation can often be recognized by a certification process. There are two MOOCs available related to AMS, from the British Society for Antimicrobial Chemotherapy with Dundee University, and Stanford University.

Clinical intelligence and big data

Clinical systems within the healthcare environment generate a huge amount of data. Clinical and business intelligence (C&BI) is the use and analysis of data captured in the healthcare setting to directly inform decision making. It has the power to make a positive impact on the delivery of patient care [8] (See Box 8.3). 'Big data' is a term applied to datasets that are so large and varied that they cannot be analysed using traditional analytical techniques. What makes data big is summarized by the three Vs: volume (the datasets are huge), velocity (the datasets are changing rapidly), and variety (the datasets contain many different types of data including structured and unstructured data). The important aspect of big data is the ability to make predictions based on the analyses. The potential for AMS is huge. An example would be integrating datasets on antibiotic use, antibiotic resistance, clinical parameters, outcome measures, and clinical notes. The future is predictive AMS!

Box 8.3 Practical points

Even without a CDSS the reporting functionality of commercial EHRs can be used to guide antimicrobial stewardship. A data warehouse (a repository of data) attached to the EHR can be interrogated using standard business intelligence tools. The use of these tools can be rapidly learnt, and most organizations will have personnel with sufficient skills for the job. This allows, for example, the AMS team to identify patients on antibiotics for review and feedback by the stewardship team, measure antimicrobial consumption, or identify missed doses.

References

1 Forrest GN, Van Schooneveld TC, Kullar R, Schulz LT, Duong P, Postelnick M. Use of electronic health records and clinical decision support systems for antimicrobial stewardship. *Clin Infect Dis* 2014;59(Suppl. 3):S122–S133.

2 HIMSS. **Electronic health records**. 2015. Available at: http://www.himss.org/library/ehr/ (accessed 25 April 2015).

3 HIMSS. *Improving outcomes with clinical decision support: an implementer's guide*. 2011. Available at: http://www.himss.org/ResourceLibrary/ResourceDetail.aspx?ItemNumber=11590 (accessed 25 March 2015).

4 Charani E, Kyratsis Y, Lawson W, Wickens H, Brannigan ET, Moore LS, et al. An analysis of the development and implementation of a smartphone application for the delivery of antimicrobial prescribing policy: lessons learnt. *J Antimicrob Chemother* 2013;68:960–7.

5 Kaplan AM, Haenlein M. Users of the world, unite! The challenges and opportunities of social media. *Business Horizons* 2010;53:59–68.

6 Goff DA, Kullar R, Newland JG. Review of Twitter for infectious diseases clinicians: useful or a waste of time? *Clin Infect Dis* 2015;60:1533–40.

7 ESGAP. **Antimicrobial stewardship virtual learning community**. 2015. Available at: http://esgap.escmid.org/?page_id=284 (accessed 20 April 2015).

8 HIMSS. **Clinical and business intelligence**. 2015. Available at: http://www.himss.org/library/clinical-business-intelligence (accessed 20 March 2015).

9 Paul M, Andreassen S, Tacconelli E, Nielsen AD, Almanasreh N, Frank U, et al. Improving empirical antibiotic treatment using TREAT, a computerized decision support system: cluster randomized trial. *J Antimicrob Chemother* 2006;58:1238–45.

10 Thursky KA, Buising KL, Bak N, Macgregor L, Street AC, Macintyre CR, et al. Reduction of broad-spectrum antibiotic use with computerized decision support in an intensive care unit. *Int J Qual Health Care* 2006;18:224–31.

11 Evans RS, Pestotnik SL, Classen DC, Clemmer TP, Weaver LK, Orme JFJr, et al. A computer-assisted management program for antibiotics and other antiinfective agents. *N Engl J Med* 1998;338:232–8.

12 Pestotnik SL, Classen DC, Evans RS, Burke JP. Implementing antibiotic practice guidelines through computer-assisted decision support: clinical and financial outcomes. *Ann Intern Med* 1996;124:884–90.

13 Calloway S, Akilo HA, Bierman K. Impact of a clinical decision support system on pharmacy clinical interventions, documentation efforts, and costs. *Hosp Pharm* 2013;48:744–52.

14 Schulz L, Osterby K, Fox B. The use of best practice alerts with the development of an antimicrobial stewardship navigator to promote antibiotic de-escalation in the electronic medical record. *Infect Control Hosp Epidemiol* 2013;34:1259–65.

15 Litvin CB, Ornstein SM, Wessell AM, Nemeth LS, Nietert PJ. Use of an electronic health record clinical decision support tool to improve antibiotic prescribing for acute respiratory infections: the ABX-TRIP study. *J Gen Intern Med* 2013;28:810–16.

Section 3

Special areas in antimicrobial stewardship

Chapter 9

Pharmacokinetic and pharmacodynamic principles of antimicrobials

Menino Osbert Cotta and Jason Roberts

Introduction to pharmacokinetic and pharmacodynamic principles of antimicrobials

Optimizing the use of antimicrobial resources is of the utmost priority in the current climate of accelerating bacterial resistance and a lack of new antibiotics.

Optimal prescribing of antimicrobials requires an understanding of the relationship between antimicrobial exposure in the body (pharmacokinetics, PK) and the corresponding clinical response (pharmacodynamics, PD). It is becoming increasingly important that antimicrobial PK/PD are taken into account when dosing antibiotics for the treatment of infections in order to ensure the maximum likelihood of clinical cure while also suppressing the emergence of antimicrobial resistance (Figure 9.1). However, challenges such as decreasing antimicrobial susceptibility and variations in PK, either by predisposition or through disease, mean that there is no 'one size fits all' approach to optimizing antimicrobial dosing. This chapter aims to summarize the principles of antimicrobial PK/PD as well as to discuss dosing implications in the setting of altered PK among specific patient populations.

Antimicrobial PK/PD indices

As the intention of antimicrobial therapy is to kill or inhibit the growth of the infective organism (described as 'kill characteristics'), the PK exposure of the antimicrobial is of paramount significance for determining the optimal dosing regimen.

The pathogen–antimicrobial exposure relationship, the PK/PD index, has been characterized in many *in vitro* and animal model studies. There are three PK/PD indices used to categorize current antimicrobials (see Figure 9.2):

(1) time dependent ($fT_{> \text{MIC}}$)

(2) concentration dependent ($C_{\text{max}}/\text{MIC}$)

(3) concentration dependent with time dependence ($\text{AUC}_{0-24}/\text{MIC}$).

All three include the main marker for antimicrobial potency, that is, the minimum inhibitory concentration (MIC) (the other terms are defined later). Identifying which PK/PD index an antimicrobial belongs to will help guide dosing strategies for optimizing therapy in the face of altered PK.

Time-dependent antimicrobials

The major killing effect of some antimicrobials relates to the time for which the unbound or 'free' concentration of the drug exceeds the MIC ($f\,T_{> \text{MIC}}$). The main antimicrobial classes that belong

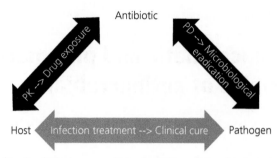

Figure 9.1 Pharmacokinetics (PK)/pharmacodynamics (PD)—relationship between antibiotic, host, and pathogen.

to this category are the β-lactams (penicillins, cephalosporins, carbapenems, and monobactams), lincosamides, and some macrolides (erythromycin and clarithromycin).

Concentration-dependent antimicrobials

For these antimicrobials the most accurate descriptor for efficacy is the ratio of the maximum antibiotic concentration (C_{max}) to the MIC (C_{max}/MIC). Antimicrobials considered to have concentration-dependent bacterial killing include aminoglycosides, fluoroquinolones, metronidazole, and lipopeptides (daptomycin).

Concentration-dependent antimicrobials with time dependence

The efficacy of some antimicrobials is best described according to the ratio of the area under the concentration–time curve during a 24-hour time period (AUC_{0-24}) to the MIC (AUC_{0-24}/MIC).

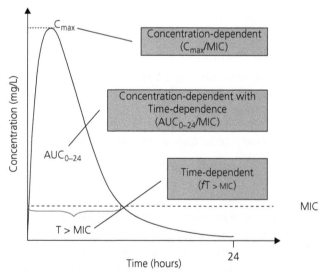

Figure 9.2 Pharmacokinetic/pharmacodynamic indices for antibiotics. Key: T > MIC, time for which the plasma concentration of the drug exceeds the minimum inhibitory concentration (MIC); $fT_{>MIC}$, time that the unbound or 'free' concentration of the drug exceeds the MIC; C_{max}/MIC, ratio of maximum antibiotic concentration (C_{max}) to the MIC; AUC_{0-24}/MIC, ratio of the area under the concentration–time curve during a 24-hour time period (AUC_{0-24}) to the MIC.

This PK/PD index is indicative of antimicrobials that display both time-dependent killing and concentration-dependent microbiological eradication. Concentration-dependent antibiotics such as aminoglycosides and fluoroquinolones, as well as time-dependent antimicrobials like linezolid, have been shown to exhibit efficacy according to AUC_{0-24}/MIC. Other antibiotics in this category include glycopeptides, tetracyclines, azithromycin, and glycylcyclines (tigecycline).

Pharmacokinetic considerations

Volume of distribution

An important aspect of the PK profile of a drug is its apparent 'volume of distribution' (Vd). The Vd is defined as the volume of fluid that a drug appears to distribute into to give it a concentration equal to that measured in plasma (Figure 9.3). Therefore, this theoretical volume provides an insight into drug distribution between the blood and the rest of the body and is determined using the following equation:

$$Vd = \frac{dose}{C_p}$$

where C_p is the concentration in plasma.

Hydrophilic antimicrobials such as β-lactams tend to concentrate more in blood and the interstitial fluid of tissues and so, as reflected by the above equation, have a smaller Vd. Conversely, non-polar or lipophilic antimicrobials, such as fluoroquinolones, tend to concentrate intracellularly as well as in adipose tissue and thus have lower measurable concentrations in blood and thus a larger Vd. The benefit of knowing the Vd of an antimicrobial is that it can guide what initial change to dosing may be required to rapidly achieve target concentrations in plasma. This may be of value when treating infections in disease states where there are significant shifts in body fluid distribution, such as severe sepsis and septic shock.

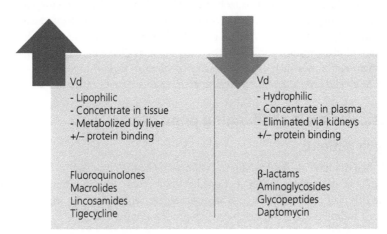

Figure 9.3 Antibiotic pharmacokinetic considerations based on volume of distribution (Vd).

Clearance

As with other drugs, the clearance (CL) of antimicrobials is an important consideration for optimizing therapy. Generally speaking, hydrophilic antimicrobials are cleared via the kidneys and so dose reductions and/or a decreasing dosing frequency should be considered to prevent accumulation of the drug and toxicity.

For time-dependent antimicrobials that are cleared via the kidneys, an appropriate dose adjustment to maintain a therapeutic exposure in renal failure may mean using lower doses rather than reducing frequency so as to maintain the PK/PD index of f $T_{> MIC}$. Predominantly renally eliminated concentration-dependent antimicrobials such as aminoglycosides, on the other hand, may require the use of a prolonged dosing interval so that C_{max}/MIC is preserved but accumulation of the drug, and the associated risk of toxicity, is minimized.

Hepatic failure can have a number of effects on the PK/PD properties of antimicrobials. Firstly, there will be an accumulation of antimicrobials metabolized and cleared by the liver and a subsequent risk of drug/metabolite accumulation and toxicity. One example of this is with the concentration-dependent antibiotic metronidazole, which is metabolized more slowly in the presence of hepatic impairment. Maintaining standard doses of 500 mg ensures that C_{max}/MIC targets are maintained, but reducing the frequency to every 12 to 24 hours in the setting of severe hepatic failure reduces the likelihood of toxic effects due to drug accumulation.

Protein binding

The affinity of antimicrobials for plasma proteins such as albumin (which constitutes approximately 60% of all plasma proteins) can affect antimicrobial activity in a number of ways. Firstly, it is the unbound or 'free' concentration of the drug that is available for distribution into extravascular spaces such as the interstitial fluid of tissues. This is an important consideration as the majority of microbial infections occur in sites other than in the blood. Additionally, only the free fraction of the drug is available for elimination from the body. Hence, CL of highly protein-bound antimicrobials via mechanisms such as tubular secretion, glomerular filtration, and hepatic metabolism can be slower than of antimicrobials with lower plasma protein-binding.

A decrease in plasma protein concentrations or a hypoalbuminaemic state (serum albumin concentrations < 25 g/L) may have dosing implications for highly protein-bound antimicrobials (>90% protein binding) such as the isoxazolyl penicillins, flucoxacillin and dicloxacillin. Although there is an increase in the unbound proportion of drug available for antibacterial activity, this is not always clinically advantageous. Rather, it can lead to enhanced CL due to higher concentrations of unbound drug, resulting in less active drug being available for antimicrobial effects. For time-dependent antibiotics such as the isoxazolyl penicillins this will mean that more frequent dosing may be a valid dose alteration to ensure maintenance of concentrations above the MIC.

Antibiotic dosing in challenging populations

Critically ill patients

Acute and often dramatic pathophysiological changes make the optimization of antibiotic dosing in the critically ill an ongoing challenge. In order to overcome these hurdles, clinicians need to evaluate the effects of critical illness, such as severe sepsis/septic shock, on the PK/PD indices of the prescribed antimicrobial using a step-by-step process (Figure 9.4).

Volume of distribution

Due to the large movements of fluid into the interstitial space as a result of endothelial dysfunction, extensive capillary leakage, and migration of albumin out of plasma (hypoalbuminaemia), one of the first PK/PD considerations is an increased Vd. Hydrophilic antimicrobials are much more affected by this fluid redistribution than lipophilic antimicrobials.

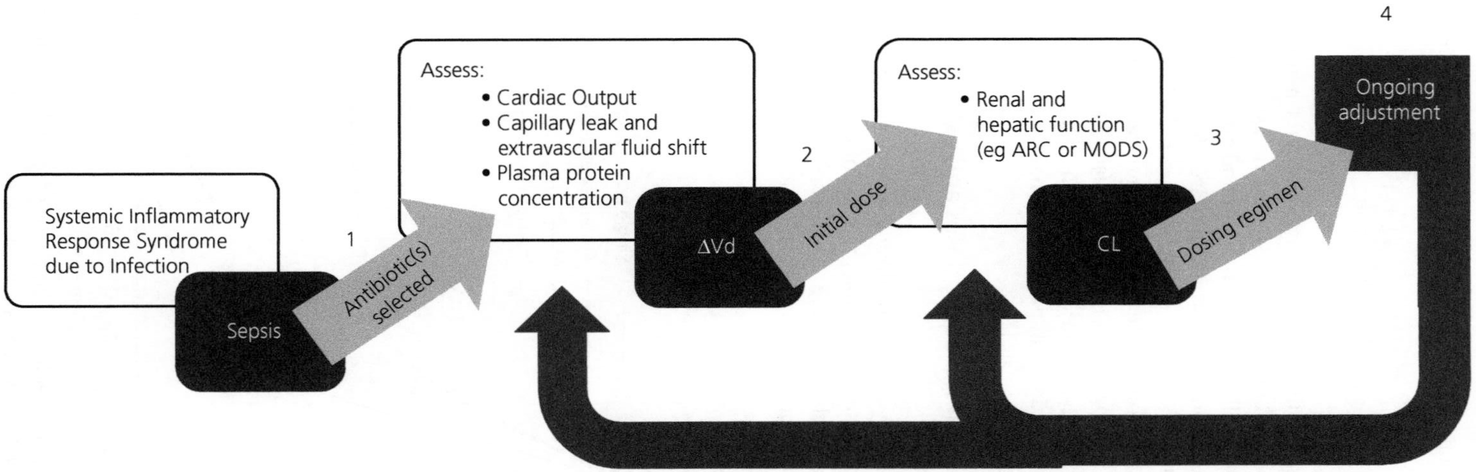

Figure 9.4 Step-wise process for antibiotic dosing in critically ill patients. Key: ARC, augmented renal clearance; CL, clearance; MODS, multiple organ dysfunction syndrome; ΔVd, change in volume of distribution.

Elimination half-life

Drug elimination is a function of both CL and Vd, as represented by the following equation:

$$t_{1/2} = \frac{0.693 \times Vd}{CL}$$

where $t_{1/2}$ is the elimination half-life. As such, $t_{1/2}$ is prolonged when Vd increases and shortened when CL increases. Sepsis-related multiple organ dysfunction syndrome (MODS), a not uncommon occurrence in the critically ill, can result in a profound extension of $t_{1/2}$ for both hydrophilic and lipophilic antimicrobials as both kidneys and liver are affected.

Conversely, some patients with sepsis may exhibit increased CL as a result of increased renal perfusion due to the administration of large amounts of intravenous fluids as well as vasopressors, leading to a decrease in $t_{1/2}$ for renally cleared antimicrobials. This increased drug CL, defined as a creatinine clearance $\geq$ 130 mL/min/1.73 m^2, has been termed 'augmented renal clearance' (ARC). It is now widely described in critically ill patients and has been associated with subtherapeutic plasma concentrations of antimicrobials [1].

Alternative dosing strategies: loading doses and extended and continuous antimicrobial infusions

In the setting of an increased Vd, standard dosing of antimicrobials is often associated with suboptimal exposure. Loading doses, therefore, may be of benefit in ensuring initial adequate concentrations of antimicrobials and have been applied for antimicrobials that have a concentration-dependent component to their efficacy, such as glycopeptides and tigecycline.

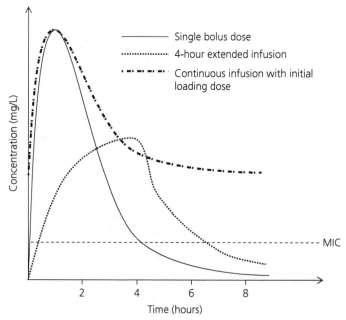

Figure 9.5 Simulated antibiotic concentration–time profiles for bolus, extended, and continuous infusions. MIC, minimum inhibitory concentration.

Higher doses of aminoglycosides among the critically ill have also been employed (e.g. ≥7 mg/kg for gentamicin and ≥25 mg/kg for amikacin, both using adjusted body weight) based on this same principle.

Increased Vd also affects how time-dependent antimicrobials are given, and dosing strategies that improve the likelihood of $fT_{> MIC}$ for 100% of the dosing interval, the ideal PK/PD index for antimicrobials such as β-lactams, may have to be employed. These include the use of more frequent administration or the use of extended (administering the antimicrobial dose over about 50% of the dosing interval) or continuous (administering the daily dose of the antibiotic as a 24-hour infusion) infusions with an initial loading dose (Figure 9.5).

Obesity

Antimicrobial dosing in the obese, defined as those with a body mass index (BMI) ≥ 30 kg/m^2, is an important consideration given the increasing prevalence of obesity worldwide. Obese patients have a higher percentage of adipose tissue and lower proportions of total body water and lean body mass than non-obese patients. As such, antimicrobial dosing strategies need to be tailored to this group of patients, paying due attention to the hydrophilicity of the antimicrobial and how it relates to body composition (i.e. the Vd of hydrophilic drugs is affected by lean body mass).

Table 9.1 Antimicrobial dosing strategies in obese patients

Antibiotic/ antibiotic class	PK/PD index	Weight used in dosing	Dosing in the obese
β-Lactams	$fT_{> MIC}$	LBW	Higher doses ± more frequent dosing, e.g. cefazolin 2 g every 4 hours
			Consider the use of extended or continuous infusions
Aminoglycosides	C_{max}/MIC	ABW	Use of TBW can lead to supratherapeutic concentrations and risk of toxicity whilst IBW does not account for the increased muscle mass which is seen in the obese
Glycopeptides	$AUC_{0–24}$/ MIC	TBW	Uncapped weight-based loading doses (15–30 mg/kg) with either intermittent or continuous infusions (if it is difficult to attain adequate trough concentrations via intermittent dosing)
Fluoroquinolones	C_{max}/MIC	ABW	Higher doses without more frequent dosing
Lincosamides	$fT_{> MIC}$	LBW	Higher doses ± more frequent dosing, e.g. clindamycin 900 mg every 6 hours
Oxazolidinones (linezolid)	$AUC_{0–24}$/ MIC	Standard dosing	Either higher doses (e.g. 1200 mg every 12 hours) or increased frequency (600 mg every 8 hours) should be considered
Lipopeptides (daptomycin)	C_{max}/MIC	LBW	Increase doses based on 4–12 mg/kg depending on indication
Glycylcyclines (tigecycline)	$AUC_{0–24}$/ MIC	Standard dosing	Consider a higher loading dose of 200 mg

Key: PK, pharmacokinetics; PD, pharmacodynamics; $fT_{> MIC}$, time that the unbound or 'free' concentration of the drug exceeds the minimum inhibitory concentration (MIC); C_{max}/MIC, ratio of maximum antibiotic concentration (C_{max}) to the MIC; $AUC_{0–24}$/MIC, ratio of the area under the concentration–time curve during a 24-hour time period ($AUC_{0–24}$) to the MIC; ABW, adjusted body weight; IBW, ideal body weight; LBW, lean body weight; TBW, total body weight.

Common weight descriptors that aid in drug dosing include total body weight (TBW), ideal body weight (IBW), adjusted body weight (ABW), and lean body weight (LBW). Interestingly, there is an increased Vd and CL for both hydrophilic and lipophilic antimicrobials in obese patients with normal renal function, so there should be due consideration given to an increase in drug dosing for both these groups of antimicrobials when optimizing dosing strategies in the obese. Of note, LBW seems to provide the best correlation with changes in Vd and CL. Table 9.1 summarizes potential strategies that may be adopted for commonly used antimicrobials and antimicrobial classes when dosing obese patients.

Conclusion

Understanding the PK/PD principles of antimicrobials represents the first step in rationalizing dosing regimens that optimize exposure to microbial pathogens. To this end, appreciation of the PK/PD index to which an antimicrobial belongs remains a fundamental consideration. Importantly, though, these bug–drug exposure relationships must take into account PK deviations among specific patient population groups, such as the critically ill and obese, so that therapy can be tailored to maximize effectiveness.

Reference

1 Udy AA, Varghese JM, Altukroni M, Briscoe S, McWhinney BC, Ungerer JP, et al. Subtherapeutic initial β-lactam concentrations in select critically ill patients: association between augmented renal clearance and low trough drug concentrations. *Chest* 2012;**142**:30–9.

Chapter 10

The role of the microbiology laboratory in antimicrobial stewardship

Peter Riley

Introduction to the role of the microbiology laboratory in antimicrobial stewardship

Microbiology laboratories play a role in antimicrobial stewardship at the individual patient and population level. When empiric therapy has been started, rapid results can lead to earlier targeted treatment. Accumulated results of susceptibility testing can be analysed and used to generate empiric treatment and prophylaxis guidelines, locally or nationally. Microbiological analysis of clinical specimens still relies on culture, but developments in differential media and the introduction of automated techniques combined with molecular methods have improved efficiency. Figure 10.1 shows the pathway of a specimen and stages where information on antimicrobial susceptibility may become available.

Organism identification and antimicrobial susceptibility testing

Accurate interpretation of the results of an antimicrobial susceptibility test (AST) requires identification of the isolate. Traditional methods rely on phenotypic properties, for example biochemical identification: this can be automated and, in some instruments, coupled with AST. Some molecular methods can be applied directly to clinical specimens. Matrix-assisted laser desorption ionization time-of-flight mass spectrometry (MALDI-TOF) is being increasingly used as the first-line test for identification [1]. With few exceptions, MALDI-TOF gives reliable identification of common bacteria and fungi, reducing the time taken for identification by 24 hours or more (e.g. identification on the same day that a blood culture becomes positive).

Choice of antibiotics to be tested

Bacterial isolates are tested against a panel of antibiotics. These are appropriate for the species (either known or predicted), the specimen site, and which antibiotics are on the hospital formulary and recommended in guidelines. Some antibiotics may not be used for treatment but are proxies for others. Further antibiotics may be tested if initial testing reveals resistance. Although all susceptibility results will be recorded, not all will be reported to the clinician (see Reporting of results).

Results are recorded in one of the following categories:

- resistant—a high likelihood of treatment failure
- susceptible—a high likelihood of treatment success
- intermediate—uncertain effect (this implies that an infection may be appropriately treated in body sites where the drugs are concentrated or when higher doses can be used).

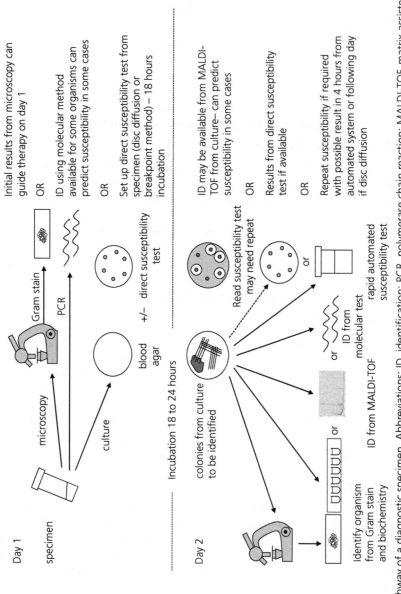

Figure 10.1 Pathway of a diagnostic specimen. Abbreviations: ID, identification; PCR, polymerase chain reaction; MALDI-TOF, matrix-assisted laser desorption ionization time-of-flight mass spectrometry.

Adapted from *Medicine*, Volume 41, Number 11, Peter A. Riley, 'Principles of microscopy, culture and serology based diagnostics', pp. 658–62, Copyright © 2013 Elsevier Ltd., with permission from Elsevier, http://www.sciencedirect.com/science/journal/13573039

Antimicrobial susceptibility tests

ASTs can be broadly divided into three groups:

1. Semi-quantitative and quantitative methods. These detect inhibition or lack of inhibition of growth of a microbe when it is exposed to an antimicrobial agent.
2. Detection of a phenotypic characteristic that predicts resistance or susceptibility.
3. Detection of a molecular characteristic that predicts resistance or susceptibility.

Table 10.1 gives details of the advantages and limitations of these different methods.

Table 10.1 Antimicrobial susceptibility tests

Susceptibility test method		Utility	Time taken for results	Direct testing on specimen	Automation	Cost*
Semi-quantitative and quantitative methods	Disc diffusion	Most organisms and antibiotics	18 hours	Possible	Limited	+
	MIC (micro/macro dilution)	Most organisms and antibiotics	4–18 hours	Limited	Possible	++
	MIC (agar incorporation)	Most organisms and antibiotics	18 hours	Possible	Possible	++
	MIC (continuous gradient disc diffusion)	Most organisms and antibiotics	18 hours	No	No	+++
Detection of a phenotypic characteristic that predicts susceptibility	Organism identity	Limited	At time of ID	Possible	Possible	+ to +++
	Detection of β-lactamase	Limited	When culture is available	No	No	+
	Detection of carbapenemase	Limited	When culture is available	No	No	+
Detection of a molecular characteristic that predicts susceptibility	PCR	Limited at present	2 hours	Possible	Possible	+++
	MALD-TOF	Limited at present	2 hours	No	No	++
	Whole genome sequencing	Limited at present	Variable	Possible	Possible	+++

* Cost relative to all methods. There may be great variation depending on the total number of tests and whether instruments are purchased or part of a reagent/rental or managed contract.

Semi-quantitative methods: disc diffusion

Disc diffusion is the most widely used method. The isolate is inoculated on semi-solid agar medium with antibiotic-impregnated discs and incubated for 18–20 hours. The diameter of the zone of inhibition of growth around the disc is measured and the bacterium is categorized as resistant, intermediate, or susceptible depending on the size of the zone and pre-defined criteria.

The zone dimensions correspond to minimum inhibitory concentrations (MICs) that have been pre-determined by testing large numbers of organisms using disc diffusion and quantitative methods in parallel [2]. Each antibiotic has a 'breakpoint' MIC for a particular bacterial species.

If the concentration needed to inhibit the bacterium is below the breakpoint, the bacterium is susceptible. If the concentration is higher than the breakpoint, the bacterium is resistant.

Many factors may influence the zone size; the medium, the size of the inoculum, temperature, atmosphere, and the duration of incubation. Most labs use a standardized approach, for example the British Society for Antimicrobial Chemotherapy (BSAC) [3] or the Clinical and Laboratory Standards Institute (CLSI) [4] methods. In Europe many individual countries have their own standards, but most are in the process of harmonizing antimicrobial breakpoints in accordance with the European Committee on Antimicrobial Susceptibility Testing (EUCAST).

In the comparative disc diffusion method the zone sizes of the test isolates are compared with those of a control inoculated on the same plate [5].

Quantitative methods: minimum inhibitory concentration

The exact concentration of an antibiotic needed to inhibit growth can be determined and is known as the MIC. The MIC may be needed for several reasons. For some species–antibiotic combinations, disc diffusion techniques are not reliable (e.g. staphylococci and glycopeptides) [3]. In some infections the MIC determines the choice and duration of treatment (e.g. the MIC of penicillin in treatment of streptococcal endocarditis) [6]. MICs are used when investigating the activity of new antimicrobials. Some laboratories use a breakpoint method for determining susceptibility for all clinical isolates.

Macro and micro broth dilution method for determining the MIC

The BSAC have published a standard method for determining the MIC [7]. Doubling dilutions of antibiotic are added to a liquid medium and this is inoculated with the test organism. The starting and finishing concentration depends on the species and the antibiotic. The method can be used in standard test tubes (macrodilution) or a microtitre plate (microdilution).

Agar dilution method

This is a useful alternative if multiple isolates need to be tested. Doubling dilutions of antibiotic are added to cooling molten agar. Standardized suspensions of bacteria are inoculated onto the plate. Multiple isolates can be tested on the same plate if a multipoint inoculator is used.

Continuous gradient disc diffusion method

This method works by establishing a concentration gradient of antibiotic on an agar plate. A commercially available form, known as the Etest [8], consists of a plastic strip that is coated on its lower surface with the antibiotic. This is placed on the inoculated plate and the antibiotic diffuses out producing a concentration gradient. The upper surface of the strip is marked with the antibiotic gradient concentrations. The MIC is read at the point that the growth (at the edge of an elliptical zone of inhibition) abuts the gradient scale. This method is easy to set up but experience is needed to read the results.

Detection of a phenotypic characteristic that predicts susceptibility

Direct β-lactamase tests are useful for *Haemophilus influenzae* and *Moraxella catarrhalis*, where only few different enzyme types occur and where enzyme production has clear implications for therapy. Chromogenic cephalosporins and acidometric or iodometric indicators are used. These rapid tests are not helpful when examining *Enterobacteriaceae* because many possible enzymes with different properties may be present. A relatively rapid spectrophotometric method that identifies carbapenamase-producing *Enterobacteriaceae* by analysing imipenem hydrolysis has been described [9].

Detection of a molecular characteristic that predicts susceptibility

Genes coding for specific enzymes or mutations that confer resistance can be detected using molecular techniques such as polymerase chain reaction (PCR) and sequencing. These methods can be applied to clinical isolates and in some circumstances directly to specimens, providing early results. Currently only a small repertoire of molecular diagnostic tests are routinely employed. These include assays to detect mutations associated with resistance in *Mycobacterium tuberculosis* and SCC*mec* in *Staphylococcus aureus* directly from specimens or on cultures, and detection of genes encoding carbapenamase enzymes in *Enterobacteriaceae* and other Gram-negative bacteria. As whole genome sequencing (WGS) becomes easier and cheaper, labs may perform sequencing to predict susceptibilities. WGS has been shown to reliably predict susceptibilities in *Mycobacterium tuberculosis* from culture [10] and directly in specimens [11] and in *S. aureus* [12], *Escherichia coli*, and *Klebsiella pneumoniae* [13]. Molecular techniques are particularly useful for mycobacteria, given the prolonged duration of culture and current phenotypic ASTs. Microengineered rapid tests that predict antimicrobial susceptibility results allowing early targeted treatment, and in the case of gonorrhoea restrict the use of cephalosporins, are under development [14].

MALDI-TOF has also been employed to predict antimicrobial susceptibility using two different approaches—changes in molecular weight that result from hydrolysis of meropenem after exposure to a bacterial isolate [15] or direct detection of up to five different β-lactamase enzymes and aminoglycoside-modifying enzymes in clinical isolates [16]. Although MALDI-TOF identification of bacteria is rapid and not technically demanding, the same is not true for demonstration of resistance. The peptide biomolecules that are markers of resistance are larger than the normal range of detection for MALD-TOF and need extraction and tryptic digestion before analysis.

Automation and early reporting of results

For disc diffusion methods, automatic plate readers can measure zone sizes. Inoculation and reading of plates can be automated for agar dilution methods. Plates containing antibiotic at the breakpoint concentration can be combined with chromogenic media allowing simultaneous identification. This is particularly useful for urine specimens where direct testing is possible. There are several commercially available automated instruments that use a microfluidic approach. Some combine AST with bacterial identification. Microtitre trays with antibiotic dilutions or small cassettes with wells are inoculated with test organisms. Turbidometric or colorimetric monitoring determines whether there is growth at the given antibiotic dilution. The organism is classified as susceptible or resistant depending on the MIC. Some instruments employ software that performs analysis of the MICs before reporting (see Reporting of results). Regular automated monitoring means that results may be available within 4 hours rather than the 18–20 hours needed for disc diffusion or agar dilution methods. Studies have demonstrated improvements in targeted therapy as well as reduced costs of further tests and shortened length of stay when automated systems are used (see Box 10.1). However, it is important to point out that benefits may not be seen in all hospitals unless there is appropriate infrastructure in place, such as extended working time in the laboratories, real-time communication of results, and staff on the wards who are available to react to the results.

Reporting of results

Expert rules

AST results need interpretation and editing before they are reported, and expert rules can be applied. EUCAST expert rules are divided into intrinsic resistance, exceptional phenotypes, and

Box 10.1 Evidence

Rapid results from the diagnostic microbiology laboratory can lead to earlier changes in antibiotic therapy

In a 1200-bed tertiary-care hospital in the Netherlands, the impact of rapid susceptibility testing and identification of positive blood cultures was compared with normal laboratory procedures [20]:

- susceptibility testing results were available 22 hours faster
- isolate identification was available 13 hours faster
- 50% of patients had their antibiotics changed to targeted therapy 1 day earlier compared with normal practice

Rapid negative results from the diagnostic microbiology laboratory can lead to earlier stopping of antibiotics

In neonatal sepsis the standard practice is for antibiotics to continue until blood cultures are negative at 48 hours. These results may only be available during the laboratory's normal working day. Many babies therefore have treatment for more than 48 hours until the result is known. In addition, there is good evidence to show that antibiotics can be safely discontinued after a negative result at 36 hours [21]. A neonatal unit at a UK maternity hospital was able to access real time results from a continuously monitored blood culture system allowing earlier decisions [22]:

- the total number of antibiotic doses administered on the unit fell from 27 700 to 16 900, an equivalent of 10 800 doses per year, or 30 doses per day based on just over 1000 admissions per year

Source: data from Keremans JJ et al. 2008 [20]; Kumar Y et al. 2001 [21]; and National Institute for Health and Care Excellence 2012 [22].

interpretive rules [17]. Ideally laboratories should employ laboratory management systems (LMS) to automatically apply these rules.

- *Intrinsic resistance*: antibiotic activity is insufficient or resistance is innate (e.g. *Enterobacteriaceae* are resistant to glycopeptides). Testing of these organism–antibiotic combinations is unnecessary but labs often test since it is more efficient to use panels or the identity of the organism is not known when the AST is set up. Some organisms may look susceptible even though the antibiotic is not considered to be active. Examples are *Enterobacteriaceae* that are known to be AmpC producers and are intrinsically resistant to co-amoxiclav.
- *Exceptional resistance*: resistance to particular antimicrobial agents that has not yet been reported or is very rare. Resistance rates change and can vary locally, nationally, and internationally, so criteria need continuous review.
- *Interpretive reading*: by reviewing the results of the susceptibility of the bacterial isolate to a range of antibiotics, the likely resistance mechanism can be predicted [18]. This allows editing of other results (see Figure 10.2).

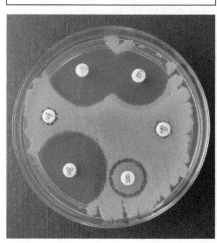

Disc diffusion antimicrobial susceptibility test for a clinical isolate of *Serratia marcescens* on Isosensitest agar and incubated at 35–37°C for 18–20 hours with the following discs; AMC30 = co-amoxiclav 30 µg, CTX30 = cefotaxime 30 µg, CN10 = gentamicin 10 µg, AML10 = amoxicillin 10 µg, CT25 = colistin 25 µg, CAZ30 = ceftazidime 30 µg.

Note resistance to colistin and co-amoxiclav, examples of intrinsic resistance for this species. Although the zone sizes of cefotaxime and ceftazidime meet the criteria for susceptible, expert rules (EUCAST) for this organism advise that because of the risk of selecting for development of resistance, use of these agents as monotherapy should be discouraged, or the results should be suppressed and not reported to the clinicians.

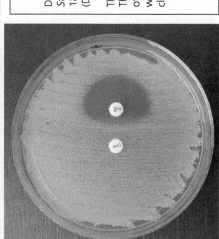

Disc diffusion antimicrobial susceptibility test for a clinical isolate of *Staphylococcus aureus* on Isosensitest agar and incubated at 35–37°C for 18–20 hours. A 5 µg erythromycin disc (E5) and a 2 µg clindamycin disc (DA2) have been placed 1.5 cm apart in the centre of the plate.

This is a test for dissociated resistance, also known as the "D test". The isolate shows no zone of inhibition to erythromycin. Note the blunting of the zone of inhibition to clindamycin. Interpretative reading of this result would conclude that the isolate has inducible resistance (MLS$_B$) to clindamycin and this agent should be used with caution or not at all.

Figure 10.2 Interpretative reading of an antimicrobial susceptibility test.

Final clinical report

After completion of AST and the application of expert rules, results should be reviewed before they are released to clinicians. Not all results will be reported (see Table 10.2). Some tests relate to antibiotics that are not in routine use, but the results of these help with the application of expert rules. For antibiotics that are used therapeutically, prescribing choices can be influenced. Most labs will only report antibiotics that correspond to the local antibiotic guidelines. The final choices of what results will be released depends on any relevant clinical information that is available. Rules can be built into LMS so that the restricted reporting happens automatically.

Table 10.2 Practical points: reporting of antimicrobial susceptibility results to prescribers

Escherichia coli **isolated from urine**	
Antibiotics tested	**Antibiotics reported to clinicians**
Amoxicillin	Yes
Co-amoxiclav	No, unless resistant to amoxicillin
Cephalexin	No, unless allergy to penicillin or resistant to amoxicillin
Cefpodoxime	No (marker for ESBL only*)
Ciprofloxacin	No unless resistant to other oral drugs or not an inpatient
	Result may also be suppressed if the patient is a child
Gentamicin	No, unless evidence of sepsis or inpatient
Trimethoprim	Yes (automatic comment if pregnant†)
Nitrofurantoin	Yes (automatic comment if pregnant†) but not reported in child < 3 months or patient with reduced eGFR

* If cefpodoxime resistant, further tests would be performed to confirm the presence of an extended spectrum β-lactamase (ESBL).

† Example of a suitable comment 'Trimethoprim should not be used in the first trimester of pregnancy. Nitrofurantoin may cause neonatal haemolysis if used at term and is therefore best avoided in the third trimester'.

With some specimens all antibiotic results may be suppressed. This happens when the isolation of an organism is of doubtful significance. The AST results will be available if, after discussion with clinicians, it is decided that treatment is needed. If treatment is not needed, the susceptibility results may still be useful for infection control purposes or for analysis of trends of antibiotic resistance.

Surveillance

AST data can be used to monitor trends in resistance locally as well as contributing to national and international surveys. Many laboratories will have LMS or other epidemiological software that allows some analysis of resistance rates for patient groups or locations (see Chapter 8). Information on local resistance rates can be provided in the form of an institutional antibiogram and fed back to prescribers.

Many countries run national surveillance schemes. In the UK, the BSAC has been running an antimicrobial resistance surveillance project since 1999 in collaboration with Public Health England (PHE) [19]. Laboratories in England also submit AST data to a national database maintained by PHE.

EARS-Net is a European network of national surveillance systems for AST data. National networks systematically collect data from laboratories in their own countries and upload the data to a central database. Denominator data on laboratory/hospital activity and patient characteristics are also collected. Since the programme began in January 1999, laboratories have collected antimicrobial resistance data on more than 400 000 invasive isolates. EARS-Net maintains an interactive database

References

1 Bizzini A, Greub G. Matrix-assisted laser desorption ionization time-of-flight mass spectrometry, a revolution in clinical microbial identification. *Clin Microbiol Infect* 2010;**16**:1614–19.

2 MacGowan AP, Wise R. Establishing MIC breakpoints and the interpretation of in vitro susceptibility tests. *J Antimicrob Chemother* 2001;**48**(Suppl. 1):17–28.

3 The British Society for Antimicrobial Chemotherapy. *BSAC methods for antimicrobial susceptibility testing*, version 14. January 2015. Available at: http://bsac.org.uk/wp-content/uploads/2012/02/BSAC-disc-susceptibility-testing-method-Jan-2015.pdf (accessed 4 March 2015).

4 Clinical and Laboratory Standards Institute (CLSI). *Performance standards for antimicrobial disk susceptibility tests; approved standard—twelfth edition*. 2012. CLSI document M02-A12. CLSI: Wayne, PA.

5 Stokes EJ, Ridgway GL, Wren MWD. *Clinical microbiology*, 7th edn, pp. 241–59, 1991. London: Edward Arnold.

6 Gould FK, Denning DW, Elliott TSJ, Foweraker J, Perry JD, Prendergast BD, et al. Guidelines for the diagnosis and antibiotic treatment of endocarditis in adults: a report of the Working Party of the British Society for Antimicrobial Chemotherapy. *J Antimicrob Chemother* 2012;**67**:269–89.

7 Andrews JM. Determination of minimum inhibitory concentrations. *J Antimicrob Chemother* 2001;**48**(Suppl. 1):5–16.

8 Bolmstrom A, Arvidson S, Ericsson M, Karisson A. A novel technique for direct quantification of antimicrobial susceptibility of microorganisms. *28th Interscience Conference on Antimicrobial Agents and Chemotherapy, Los Angeles, USA, 1988.* Abstract 1209.

9 Bernabeu S, Poirel L, Nordmann P. Spectrophotometry-based detection of carbapenemase producers among Enterobacteriaceae. *Diag Microbiol Infect Dis* 2010;**74**:88–90.

10 Köser CU, Bryant JM, Becq J, Török ME, Ellington MJ, Marti-Renom MA, et al. Whole-genome sequencing for rapid susceptibility testing of *M. tuberculosis*. *New Engl J Med* 2013;**369**:290–2.

11 Witney AA, Gould KA, Arnold A, Coleman D, Delgado R, Dhillon J, et al. Clinical application of whole genome sequencing to inform treatment for multi-drug resistant tuberculosis cases. *J Clin Microbiol* 2015;**53**:1473–83.

12 Gordon NC, Price JR, Cole K, Everitt R, Morgan M, Finney J, et al. Prediction of *Staphylococcus aureus* antimicrobial resistance by whole-genome sequencing. *J Clin Microbiol* 2014;**52**:1182–91.

13 Stoesser N, Batty EM, Eyre DW, Morgan M, Wyllie DH, Del Ojo Elias C, et al. Predicting antimicrobial susceptibilities for *Escherichia coli* and *Klebsiella pneumoniae* isolates using whole genomic sequence data. *J Antimicrob Chemother* 2013;**68**:2234–44.

14 Sadiq ST, Dave J, Butcher PD. Point-of-care antibiotic susceptibility testing for gonorrhoea: improving therapeutic options and sparing the use of cephalosporins. *Sex Transm Infect* 2010;**86**:445–6.

15 Hrabák J, Walková R, Studentová V, Chudácková E, Bergerová T. Carbapenemase activity detection by matrix-assisted laser desorption ionization-time of flight mass spectrometry. *J Clin Microbiol* 2011;**49**:3222–7.

16 Hart PJ, Wey E, McHugh TJ, Balakrishnan I, Belqacem O. A method for the detection of antibiotic resistance markers in clinical strains of *Escherichia coli* using MALDI mass spectrometry. *J Microbiol Methods* 2015;**111**:1–8.

17 Leclercq R, Cantón R, Brown DF, Giske CG, Heisig P, MacGowan AP, et al. EUCAST expert rules in antimicrobial susceptibility testing. *Clin Microbiol Infect* 2013;**19**:141–60.

18 Livermore DM, Winstanley TG, Shannon KP. Interpretative reading: recognizing the unusual and inferring resistance mechanisms from resistance phenotypes. *J Antimicrob Chemother* 2001;**48**(Suppl. 1):87–102.

19 **Reynolds R, Hope R** and **Williams L** on behalf of the BSAC Working Parties on Resistance Surveillance. Survey, laboratory and statistical methods for the BSAC resistance surveillance programmes. *J Antimicrob Chemother* 2008;**62**(Suppl. 2):ii15–ii28.

20 **Kerremans JJ, Verboom P, Stijnen T, Hakkaart-van Roijen L, Goessens W, Verbrugh HA, et al.** Rapid identification and antimicrobial susceptibility testing reduce antibiotic use and accelerate pathogen-directed antibiotic use. *J Clin Microbiol* 2008;**61**:428–35.

21 **Kumar Y, Qunibi M, Neal TJ, Yoxall CW.** Time to positivity of neonatal blood cultures. *Arch Dis Child Fetal Neonatal Ed* 2001;**85**:F182–F186.

22 **National Institute for Health and Care Excellence.** Supporting a 36 hour neonatal blood culture status check by developing the availability of blood culture status in real time. June 2012. Available at: https://www.nice.org.uk/sharedlearning/supporting-a-36-hour-neonatal-blood-culture-status-check-by-developing-the-availability-of-blood-culture-status-in-real-time (accessed 26 January 2016).

Chapter 11

Antimicrobial stewardship in the immunocompromised patient

Haifa Lyster

Introduction to antimicrobial stewardship in the immunocompromised patient

Antibiotic resistance is a critically important issue for immunocompromised patients, who depend on rapid treatment with active antibiotics for survival. Advances in the management of cancer, solid organ transplantation (SOT), and haematopoietic stem-cell transplantation (HSCT) have improved survival while immunomodulating therapies have reduced morbidity in immunological disorders such as rheumatoid arthritis and inflammatory bowel disease. These advances in medical care are being jeopardized by the emergence of highly resistant infections in this group of patients [1,2]. Such resistance is largely driven by repeated and often prolonged use of broad-spectrum antimicrobials [3]. Thus, it is crucial that antimicrobial stewardship (AMS) is implemented effectively in immunocompromised patients.

The stewardship strategies detailed in Chapters 5–8 are valid in immunocompromised patients. However, there are a number of challenges to this process; most notably, immunocompromised patients are susceptible to a broad spectrum of infections that can progress rapidly. This is usually at the forefront of a clinician's mind when initiating or reviewing antibiotic therapy and can cause conflict with some stewardship strategies.

Principles of AMS in an immuncompromised host

Gyssens et al. [2] have developed a specific set of AMS principles for haematology patients, the majority of which are applicable to other groups of immunosuppressed patients (Box 11.1).

The evidence to support implementation of antimicrobial stewardship programmes (ASPs) in immunocompromised patient groups is scarce compared with that in the general population, and this is an issue that needs to be addressed. ASPs in cancer patients have largely focused on reducing the time to first antibiotic dose in neutropenic sepsis, which has been associated with lower mortality rates [4]. An ASP in hospitalized HIV patients has been shown to reduce medication errors [5]. There are currently no AMS guidelines for SOT patients [6].

Net state of immunosuppression

The concept of 'net state of immunosuppression' is complex and is a combination of immunosuppressive agents, neutropenia, and malnutrition, as well as infections with immunomodulating viruses such as HIV. It can vary between patients and there is intrapatient variability over time. For example, transplant patients are on a multidrug regimen of immunosuppressants with higher doses during the early period post-SOT when the risk of rejection is greatest.

Box 11.1 Principles of AMS in the immunocompromised host

- Guidance on the diagnosis, treatment, and prophylaxis of fever during neutropenia should be developed and should include advice on duration of therapy for the inpatient as well as outpatient management

- Empiric antibiotic therapy should be prompted by fever and clinical signs, as studies have shown inconsistent results with the use of biomarkers

- Antibiotics should not be initiated on the basis of colonization by resistant organisms

- Empiric therapy should not be initiated or escalated before taking appropriate cultures (at least two blood cultures in addition to relevant specimens from clinical sites of infection)

- Risk stratification for infection should be undertaken according to the Multinational Association for Supportive Care in Cancer (MASCC) score, and should be considered in treatment guidelines

- Empiric therapy should, at the very least, cover common virulent *Enterobacteriaceae*, *Pseudomonas aeruginosa*, and, *Staphylococcus aureus*

- Individualized risk assessment for multiresistant pathogens should guide the development of treatment algorithms.

- Strategies to reassess empiric antibiotic therapy after 2–3 days should be implemented, with de-escalation where possible

- Epidemiological data on blood isolates and colonization should be examined on a regular basis

- Infection-related outcome data (length of stay, infection-related mortality) should be monitored

- Microbiology, antibiotic use, and outcome data should be discussed in local multidisciplinary team meetings consisting of the parent team (e.g. haematologists), infectious disease (ID) specialists, and/or microbiologists and ID pharmacists

- ID training for should be provided for the parent team (e.g. haematologists) and clinical training for ID physicians/microbiologists and pharmacists in the area in which they will perform stewardship

- Individualized risk assessments for infection can be undertaken considering the net state of immunosuppression

Adapted with permission from Inge C. et al., on behalf of ECIL-4, a joint venture of EBMT, EORTC, ICHS and ESGICH of ESCMID, 'The role of antibiotic stewardship in limiting antibacterial resistance among hematology patients,' *Haematologica*, Volume 98, Number 12, pp. 1821–25, Copyright © 2013 Ferrata Storti Foundation.

Challenges for stewardship in the immunocompromised host

Physician perceptions and attitudes

The perceptions and attitudes of the team of physicians looking after immunocompromised patients are important factors for successful AMS (see Chapter 3): in a survey to assess attitudes, perceptions, and knowledge, about antimicrobial use and resistance physicians said that their antibiotic prescribing was most influenced by the risk of missing an infection and whether a patient was critically ill or immunosuppressed [7]. This means that broad-spectrum antimicrobials are often prescribed for extended periods of time and de-escalation or discontinuation of antimicrobials is resisted by clinicians as these patients are deemed 'sicker' than immunocompetent patients.

AMS is a multidisciplinary team approach; to work effectively there should be close collaboration between the antimicrobial management team (AMT) and the parent team with a shared appreciation of the complexities of caring for these patients. A consistent AMT is important to increase compliance and acceptance and develop trust. Dedicated consultant-level clinicians should play a crucial role in ASPs in this setting [8] because junior team members are not empowered to, or do not have sufficient confidence to, discontinue antimicrobial therapy.

Diagnostics

Diagnosing 'proven' infection is challenging in immunocompromised patients due to the effects of immunosuppressant treatment and host factors, which may dampen clinical signs and symptoms of infection. Certain diagnostic procedures may also prove challenging in this patient group; patients may, for example, be too unwell for imaging or have contra-indications to invasive sampling such as biopsies. Further complications could include presentation with mixed infections or colonization by a number of potential pathogens, which must be accurately differentiated from active or invasive disease.

The facilitation of rapid and accurate diagnostics can support AMS, hence a close link with the microbiology laboratory is essential (see Chapters 10 and 17).

Neutropenic sepsis—the golden hour!

The National Institute for Health and Care Excellence (NICE) guideline on the prevention and management of neutropenic sepsis in cancer patients aims to 'improve outcomes by providing evidence-based recommendations on the prevention, identification and management of life-threatening complications of cancer treatment' [9]. A number of recommendations pose difficulties in application, particularly the 1 hour time to administration of the first dose of antibiotics. A national audit highlighted that this standard was achieved in only 26% of patients [10]. The most common reasons for the delay were that the administration of the antibiotic was delayed by nurses following prompt prescribing or there was a prolonged time to assessment by a junior doctor [10]. There are a number of strategies employed to improve this, such as introducing local 'patient group directives' allowing trained nurses to initiate treatment without a doctor's signature, increasing awareness of the importance of the 1-hour target, and not waiting for blood results prior to administering the antibiotic.

De-escalation

De-escalation is a particular challenge in the immunocompromised host, due to both physician beliefs and the difficulties in diagnostics already detailed. However, it is a critically important AMS strategy because immunocompromised patients are likely to develop frequent infections and receive repeated courses of antimicrobial therapy in a relatively short period of time, often on the background of prolonged antimicrobial prophylaxis. This practice has been associated with the emergence of resistant pathogens, particularly among Gram-negative bacilli [11], with carbapenem-resistant *Enterobacteriaceae* being a major concern [1,2] as mortality rates with such infections are 40% in SOT recipients and 65% in patients with haematological malignancies [12].

There is evidence to show that de-escalation can be accomplished safely in this patient group: three studies of patients with neutropenic sepsis have shown early de-escalation from intravenous broad-spectrum treatment to oral prophylaxis to be safe where evidence of infection was lacking, even when patients remained neutropenic [13–15].

The ECIL-4 guideline on empiric antibacterial therapy for febrile neutropenic patients supports such a strategy, suggesting that for stable patients who are afebrile for more than 48 hours and have no microbiological or clinical documentation of infection the treatment duration should be limited to 72 hours [16].

A further study supports the safety and efficacy of de-escalating from broad-spectrum to narrow targeted therapy in microbiologically confirmed infection, as guided by antimicrobial susceptibility testing [11]

Pharmacokinetics/pharmacodynamics

Optimization of pharmacokinetics/pharmacodynamics is crucially important in patients with malfunctioning immune systems and those whose pathogens have only borderline antibiotic susceptibility [17]. Detailed information on how to optimize therapy is given in Chapter 9.

Drug interactions and co-morbidities

Formulary review of antimicrobial agents taking into account their efficacy, adverse effects, and costs as well as patients' common co-morbidities, for example renal impairment and bone marrow suppression, should go in parallel with the development of institutional clinical guidelines. Highly active antiretroviral therapy (HAART) and immunosuppressants are associated with significant drug–drug interactions—multidisciplinary stewardship efforts can reduce medication errors in these patient groups with pharmacists playing a major role [5,18].

Fungi and viruses

While AMS usually refers to antibiotics, in immunosuppressed patients AMS should also include antifungal and antiviral therapies. Antifungal stewardship is discussed in Chapter 16. Consensus guidelines on the management of opportunistic viral infections are lacking, which makes antiviral stewardship a challenging and neglected field at present.

Conclusions

Caring for immunocompromised patients is challenging, and infection is a major cause of morbidity and mortality. There is a need for AMS as it can have a positive impact on limiting the prevalence of infections with multidrug-resistant organisms. Collaboration with local experts and the use of early diagnostic testing are both essential for a successful ASP.

References

1 Satlin MJ, Jenkins SG, Walsh TJ. The global challenge of carbapenem-resistant Enterobacteriaceae in transplant recipients and patients with hematologic malignancies. *Clin Infect Dis* 2014;**58**:1274–83.

2 Gyssens IC, Kern WV, Livermore DM; on behalf of ECIL-4, a joint venture of EBMT, EORTC, ICHS and ESGICH of ESCMID. The role of antibiotic stewardship in limiting antibacterial resistance among hematology patients. *Haematologica* 2013;**98**:1821–5.

3 Gudiol C, Tubau F, Calatayud L, Garcia-Vidal C, Cisnal M, Sanchez-Ortega I, et al. Bacteraemia due to multidrug-resistant Gram-negative bacilli in cancer patients: risk factors, antibiotic therapy and outcomes. *J Antimicrob Chemother* 2011;**66**:657–63.

4 Rosa RG, Goldani LZ, dos Santos RP. Association between adherence to an antimicrobial stewardship program and mortality among hospitalised cancer patients with febrile neutropaenia: a prospective cohort study. *BMC Infect Dis* 2014;**14**:286.

5 **Sanders J, Pallotta A, Bauer S, Sekeres J, Davis R, Taege A, et al.** Antimicrobial stewardship program to reduce antiretroviral medication errors in hospitalized patients with human immunodeficiency virus infection. *Infect Control Hosp Epidemiol* 2014;**35**:272–7.

6 **Aitken SL, Palmer HR, Topal JE, Gabardi S, Tichy E.** Call for antimicrobial stewardship in solid organ transplantation. *Am J Transplant* 2013;**13**:2499.

7 **Abbo L, Sinkowitz-Cochran R, Smith L, Ariza-Heredia E, Gomez-Marin O, Srinivasan A, et al.** Faculty and resident physicians' attitudes, perceptions, and knowledge about antimicrobial use and resistance. *Infect Control Hosp Epidemiol* 2011;**32**:714–18.

8 **Yeo CL, Wu JE, Chung GW-T, Chan DS-G, Fisher D, Hsu LY.** Specialist trainees on rotation cannot replace dedicated consultant clinicians for antimicrobial stewardship of specialty disciplines. *Antimicrob Resist Infect Control* 2012;**1**:36.

9 **Bate J, Gibson F, Johnson E, Selwood K, Skinner R, Chisholm J.** Neutropenic sepsis: prevention and management of neutropenic sepsis in cancer patients (NICE Clinical Guideline CG151). *Arch Dis Child Educ Pract Ed* 2013;**98**:73–5.

10 **Clarke RT, Warnick J, Stretton K, Littlewood TJ.** Improving the immediate management of neutropenic sepsis in the UK: lessons from a national audit. *Br J Haematol* 2011;**153**:773–9.

11 **Rolston KV, Mahajan SN, Chemaly RF.** Antimicrobial de-escalation in cancer patients. *Infection* 2012;**40**:223–4.

12 **Johnson K, Boucher HW.** Editorial commentary: imminent challenges: carbapenem-resistant enterobacteriaceae in transplant recipients and patients with hematologic malignancy. *Clin Infect Dis* 2014;**58**:1284–6.

13 **De Marie S, Van den Broek PJ, Willemze R, Van Furth R.** Strategy for antibiotic therapy in febrile neutropenic patients on selective antibiotic decontamination. *Eur J Clin Microbiol Infect Dis* 1993;**12**:897–906.

14 **Cornelissen JJ, Rozenberg-Arska M, Dekker AW.** Discontinuation of intravenous antibiotic therapy during persistent neutropenia in patients receiving prophylaxis with oral ciprofloxacin. *Clin Infect Dis* 1995;**21**:1300–2.

15 **Slobbe L, Waal L, Jongman LR, Lugtenburg PJ, Rijnders BJ.** Three-day treatment with imipenem for unexplained fever during prolonged neutropaenia in haematology patients receiving fluoroquinolone and fluconazole prophylaxis: a prospective observational safety study. *Eur J Cancer* 2009;**45**:2810–17.

16 **Averbuch D, Orasch C, Cordonnier C, Livermore DM, Mikulska M, Viscoli C, et al.; on behalf of ECIL4, a joint venture of EBMT, EORTC, ICHS, ESGICH/ESCMID and EL.** European guidelines for empirical antibacterial therapy for febrile neutropenic patients in the era of growing resistance: summary of the 2011 4th European Conference on Infections in Leukemia. *Haematologica* 2013;**98**:1826–35.

17 **Abbott IJ, Roberts JA.** Infusional beta-lactam antibiotics in febrile neutropenia: has the time come? *Curr Opin Infect Dis* 2012;**25**:619–25.

18 **Eginger KH, Yarborough LL, Inge LD, Basile SA, Floresca D, Aaronson PM.** Medication errors in HIV-infected hospitalized patients: a pharmacist's impact. *Ann Pharmacother* 2013;**47**:953–60.

Chapter 12

Antimicrobial stewardship in the intensive care setting

Jonathan Ball

Introduction to antimicrobial stewardship in the intensive care setting

The principles and interventions of antimicrobial stewardship (AMS) hold true for, and are especially important in, critically ill patients.

Critically ill patients are those with acute, severe, and potentially life-threatening organ dysfunction and/or failure. Placing such patients in specialist ward areas evolved slowly as a consequence of the development of continuous physiological monitoring and organ supportive therapies, both mechanical and pharmacological, during the 1950s and 1960s. The successful delivery of care to the critically ill involves a large, specialist, multidisciplinary team including doctors, nurses, allied healthcare professions, and supporting services.

Intensive care units

Commonly referred to as intensive or critical care units (ICUs) such wards vary significantly in terms of:

- size
- patient population: neonatal, paediatric, adult, mixed; general/mixed verses organ-specific/specialist, e.g. cardiac, cardiothoracic, neurology/neurosurgery, liver, burns
- physical environment: old verses new; open plan verses single rooms; co-location with other ward environments
- delivery of care models: open versus closed; 1:1 verses team nursing; etc.

In short, there is considerable heterogeneity between units.

Regardless of these differences, all ICUs frequently care for patients with life-threatening infections and thus harbour reservoirs of pathogenic microorganisms. Furthermore, as a direct consequence of their critical illness/injury, ICU patients commonly have a significant degree of acutely acquired, innate, and adaptive immune system dysfunction. Added to this, they have often lost normal barrier defences and are immobile and dysglycaemic with tissue/organ hypoperfusion. Thus, critically ill patients have an increased susceptibility to colonization and infection with common, atypical, and even opportunistic pathogens. As a consequence, the use of broad-spectrum antimicrobials, as both empiric and targeted therapy, is common, creating a selection pressure within both the patient and the environment. Viewed as a microbiology experiment, ICUs create an ideal environment for the selection, amplification, and dissemination of resistant organisms. Accordingly, there are obvious benefits from AMS, both to optimize effective care and as a component of infection control policy within ICUs.

In order to discuss the components of AMS in the ICU, in the following sections we shall consider two broad clinical scenarios.

Primary acute severe infection causing critical illness

Infections cause critical illness by inducing severe isolated organ dysfunction, a secondary multiple organ dysfunction (sepsis) syndrome, or both. The most common causative organisms are bacteria. Common primary sites include the lower respiratory tract, the urinary tract, the bilary tract, the peritoneum, skin/soft tissues, and the meninges. The PIRO model (Predisposition, Infection, Response, Organ dysfunction) [1] is a helpful conceptual tool:

- predisposition of the patient: extremes of age, acute co-morbidities, chronic diseases/therapies, genetics
- infection: virulence factors in the causative organism
- response: measurable physiological and biochemical makers that correlate with the severity of illness
- organ dysfunction: the degree of individual organ dysfunction, which may be entirely acute or acute on chronic.

Patients may acquire such infections either spontaneously in the community or as a complication of an acute illness or surgery. The epidemiology of such infections has been well described. They are very common and associated with both a high risk of mortality and long-term morbidity in survivors. Early recognition of sepsis is important, because the earlier effective systemic antibiotics are administered (and, where applicable, source control can be achieved) the better the outcome. The realization of the burden of these diseases and the proven efficacy of time-critical interventions has resulted in national and international campaigns to raise awareness, create early recognition tools, and promote best practice/evidenced-based timely interventions [2,3]. However, these efforts are hampered by two distinct problems. First, there can be significant difficulty in confirming the specific diagnosis, most especially identifying the causative organism and its susceptibility to specific antibiotics. The second problem relates to on-going controversies about the value and timing of specific interventions. Current consensus dictates the following: in the setting of an acute severe illness, in which an infective aetiology is a reasonable probability, blood and any other appropriate and easily accessible bodily fluid/tissue should be obtained for microbiological laboratory investigations followed by administration of a broad-spectrum, empiric, systemic antibiotic. These actions should be prioritized over all but immediate life-saving interventions. As such, they should occur before a patient is admitted to an ICU.

In terms of antibiotic stewardship the clinical imperatives of not wanting to miss the possibility of a serious infection and the time-critical administration of broad-spectrum systemic antibiotics present significant challenges.

Successful strategies that can be employed to optimize the initiation of antibiotic therapy are:

- The use of these clinical imperatives to ensure/persuade that senior clinicians are involved in refining the diagnosis and prioritizing the care of such patients, at the earliest opportunity. This should include, where indicated, timely referral to the ICU. Make expert advice from medical infection specialists readily available and encourage this dialogue.
- Conduct regular local campaigns regarding the value of, and the best techniques for obtaining, microbiology specimens. Include feedback on recent cases, preferably known to, or relevant to, the team.

- Link the acquisition of microbiology specimens with the prescription and administration of empiric antibiotics and with clinical documentation.

- Create, publicize, and police a local empiric antibiotic guideline that covers all common clinical scenarios. Embed details of the guideline into all local induction processes.

- Subject the guideline to regular audit and periodic (annual) review, both of which present a useful opportunity to re-publicize the guideline.

- The periodic review should consider any changes in the spectrum of pathogens or patterns of antibiotic resistance. This obviously requires the routine collection and analysis of longitudinal data specific to the unit/area/hospital to which the guideline applies. The review should be conducted as a collaboration between frontline clinicians, medical infection specialists, and specialist pharmacists. A mechanism should exist to facilitate a change to the guideline in response to the sudden emergence of a new pathogen or antibiotic resistance pattern outside of the planned periodic review.

Secondary acute severe infection complicating a critical illness

As mentioned in the Introduction, critically ill patients are very vulnerable to the acquisition of secondary infections. Common clinical scenarios are detailed in Table 12.1. As with primary infections, these can cause both local and systemic problems. These infections can be very challenging to diagnose as all of the non-specific clinical and laboratory signs of sepsis, pyrexia, tachycardia, increasing total white blood cell count, neutrophil count, and C-reactive protein (CRP) often have more probable, non-infective explanations. These might include the development of a new, or progression of an existing, inflammatory pathology or recent surgery. To complicate matters further, secondary infections are more likely than primary infections to be due to resistant bacteria, environmental pathogens, fungi, or viruses. Accordingly, though the basic tenets of culture and timely administration of empiric therapy still stand, the more complex clinical circumstances need to be taken into account.

Differences in approach include:

- Patients are often already receiving, or have recently completed, courses of prophylactic or therapeutic antibiotics. This may adversely affect the isolation of active pathogens.

- There is increasing evidence that the pharmacokinetics of antimicrobials are significantly altered in many critically ill patients. This may result is enhanced clearance such that treatment failures occur. As therapeutic drug monitoring is only routinely available for a tiny minority of agents, empiric dosing schedules for specific agents based upon individual patient circumstances are required. Unavoidably, this adds substantially to the complexity of empiric guidelines [4].

- Blood cultures taken from indwelling lines may yield false positive results, thus a peripheral sample should always be taken. The value of simultaneous cultures from lines is debated.

- As regards source control, whether or not a vascular access device should be removed and/or replaced before the diagnosis of catheter-related bloodstream infection is confirmed may require careful consideration of the pros and cons.

- Imaging can be invaluable in refining the differential diagnosis, but repeated whole-body CT scans conducted as 'fishing expeditions' for occult infection carry a heavy burden in terms of exposure to ionizing radiation.

- By necessity, empiric therapy needs to be broader and is likely to include two or more agents.

Table 12.1 Common secondary acute severe infections complicating a critical illness

Organ system	Common clinical scenarios	Specific predisposing factors	Specific preventative and reactive interventions	Controversies
Respiratory	Hypostatic pneumonia Ventilator-associated infection—a broad spectrum encompassing respiratory tract colonization, tracheobronchitis, and pneumonia	Immobility and recumbent positioning Altered level of consciousness ± sedative medication Instrumented upper airway Positive pressure ventilation Impaired mucocillary escalator and cough Altered airway surface liquid Lung atelectasis Oropharyngeal colonization and mircoaspiration Gastric acid suppression	Regular repositioning Minimize sedation and ensure at least daily cessation Active weaning programme including de-escalation to less invasive support Optimize airway hydration Routine oral hygiene regime	Value of maintaining minimum 30° head-up position Optimal sedation strategies Optimal weaning strategies Optimal method of airway hydration Value of specialist airway tubes—including subglottic suction ports Value of selective oral and upper gastrointestinal tract decontamination
Cardiovascular	Catheter-related bloodstream infections Infective endocarditis	The need for intravascular catheters for invasive monitoring and delivery of care	Aseptic insertion and avoidance of the femoral site Aseptic handling Dedicated lumens for parenteral nutrition Daily review of ongoing need with removal at the earliest opportunity	Specialist coatings for catheters Regular periodic change
Gastrointestinal tract	Antibiotic-associated diarrhoea *Clostridium difficile* colitis Acalculus cholecystitis and ascending cholangitis	Broad-spectrum antibiotic therapy Gastric acid suppression Cholestasis	Antibiotic stewardship Early institution of enteral feeding	Probiotics Recolonization strategies

(*continued*)

Table 12.1 Continued

Organ system	Common clinical scenarios	Specific predisposing factors	Specific preventative and reactive interventions	Controversies
Renal	Urinary catheter-related infection—a spectrum encompassing colonization, local symptoms, and sepsis	The need to manage urinary drainage in patients unable to manage this task for themselves Diarrhoea—multifactorial, most commonly functional	Aseptic insertion Aseptic handling Daily review of ongoing need with removal at the earliest opportunity	Interpretation of urine specimens obtained from an indwelling catheter
Central nervous system	Ventriculitis	The clinical need for external ventricular drainage	Prophylactic intrathecal antibiotics	Value and safety of prophylaxis?
Skin and soft tissues	Surgical site/wound infection	Dysglycaemia Use of vasopressors Tissue oedema		
Body cavities	Sinusitis Empyema Spontaneous bacterial peritonitis	Nasal tubes and artificial airways Positive pressure ventilatory support and positive cumulative fluid balance Acute, or acute on chronic, liver injury		

AMS in these circumstances is especially challenging and a variety of successful strategies should be considered [3,5].

Daily infection rounds should be conducted, comprising senior frontline clinicians (intensive care medicine specialists and ideally any and all other specialists involved in the patient's care), medical infection specialists, and specialist pharmacists. These can be embedded into the unit's daily rounds or occur separately. The value of making the intensive care medicine specialist the final arbiter of diagnosis and decision to start or switch antimicrobial therapy is arguably best practice, and it is important that they weigh up competing advice and priorities from the differing teams.

Specialists in intensive care should adopt working patterns that maximize the continuity of care for intensive care patients. Typically this involves duty periods of a week. Making one of the team of intensive care specialists responsible for the oversight of AMS is valuable. Having medical infection specialists and pharmacists dedicated to individual units has obvious benefits.

For antimicrobials whose efficacy is time dependent, routine administration should entail a loading dose followed by continuous infusion. A high-dose, minimum-duration strategy should be employed.

After '48 hours', negative cultures, taken in the context of the patient's clinical trajectory/responsive to empiric antimicrobial therapy, should result in active consideration of the cessation of the antimicrobial. Positive cultures should result in the re-evaluation of any and all source control interventions, such as removal of potentially colonized devices, and narrowing the spectrum of therapy.

Clinical response parameters should be set for stopping therapy. These should include both clinical resolution and serial inflammatory markers. Of these, CRP is probably the best of the readily available markers. One threshold identified as a potential stopping criterion is a CRP level of less than 50% of the peak level. Given the known lag in the kinetics of CRP, this probably represents an 'extra 24 hours' of antimicrobial therapy. Procalcitonin-based strategies are discussed in Chapter 17.

A concise weekly report of all positive cultures of patients admitted to an ICU should be sent to all senior clinicians. This should alert them to any emerging patterns that might influence clinical decisions or highlight a potential failure of routine infection control practices.

Interventions such as antimicrobial guidelines, education, and computer decision support tools are discussed elsewhere in this book.

The screening of ICU patients for the carriage of commonly occurring resistant bacteria is commonly practised but is of uncertain benefit. The value of regular screening of high-risk areas within the ICU is also controversial. However, if it identifies a reservoir of potential pathogens remedial interventions can be undertaken. A periodic or persistent problem may require changes to second- or even firstline empiric therapy [6].

Even with the use of rapid diagnostics there is an inevitable delay in identifying carriers. Thus the only safe and sustainable solution is the routine use of a universal precautions approach to infection control. Some units have included in their approach the provision of single-room-only ICUs, all of which have individually controllable airflow and HEPA filtration. However, the additional costs of construction and running such a unit are significant. Furthermore, there is a growing body of evidence that single-room-only designs result in a significant reduction in the overall quality of care delivered. Finally, there are many examples of open plan units with consistently zero levels of cross-infection between patients, thus demonstrating the lack of efficacy of the single-room-only approach.

If the hospital population as a whole or a specific, easily identifiable group has a significant level of asymptomatic colonization of a resistant organism then this must be accounted for in empiric antibiotic guidelines. If the screening programme reveals a sudden cluster of colonized and/or infected patients then remedial interventions can be considered, including enhanced environmental cleaning, review of adherence to infection control practices, and consideration of the pros and cons of moving patients into a more stringent isolated environment.

References

1 **Marshall JC.** The PIRO (predisposition, insult, response, organ dysfunction) model: toward a staging system for acute illness. *Virulence* 2014;5: 27–35.

2 **Cohen J, Vincent JL, Adhikari NK, Machado FR, Angus DC, Calandra T, et al.** Sepsis: a roadmap for future research. *Lancet Infect Dis* 2015;15:581–614.

3 **Society of Critical Care Medicine.** Surviving sepsis campaign: guidelines. 2012. Available at: http://www.survivingsepsis.org/guidelines/Pages/default.aspx (accessed 15 March 2015).

4 **Blot SI, Pea F, Lipman J.** The effect of pathophysiology on pharmacokinetics in the critically ill patient—concepts appraised by the example of antimicrobial agents. *Adv Drug Deliv Rev* 2014;77:3–11.

5 **Zhang YZ, Singh S.** Antibiotic stewardship programmes in intensive care units: why, how, and where are they leading us. *World J Crit Care Med* 2015;4:13–28.

6 **Landelle C, Marimuthu K, Harbarth S.** Infection control measures to decrease the burden of antimicrobial resistance in the critical care setting. *Curr Opin Crit Care* 2014;20:499–506.

Chapter 13

Surgical prophylaxis

Tamsin Oswald, Simon Jameson, and Mike Reed

Introduction to surgical prophylaxis

Infections that occur in the wound created by an invasive surgical procedure are generally referred to as surgical site infections (SSIs). SSIs are one of the most important causes of healthcare-associated infections (HCAIs). A prevalence survey reported that SSIs account for 14% of HCAIs, and nearly 5% of patients who had undergone a surgical procedure were found to have developed a SSI [1].

SSIs are associated with considerable morbidity, and it has been reported that over a third of post-operative deaths are related to one SSI [2]. The survival rate of an infected joint replacement is 87.3% at 5 years [3]. A SSI can double the length of hospital stay, thereby increasing healthcare costs. Additional costs attributable to SSIs of between £814 and £100 000 have been reported depending on the type of surgery and the severity of the infection [4–6].

SSI is multifactorial involving patient, surgical, and environmental factors. Although this chapter will focus on the use of antibiotics for prophylaxis there are many key interventions to reduce infections for patients undergoing surgery, and thus the subsequent need for treatment with antibiotics. These interventions include: optimization of diabetes, reducing obesity and smoking, meticulous surgical site preparation, patient warming, theatre design, personnel clothing, oxygen therapy, goal-directed fluid therapy, and avoidance of blood transfusion [7–9]. Introducing SSI surveillance has been shown to significantly reduce infection rates and save healthcare costs [10]. The surveillance teams collect accurate and credible data, which should be used to drive proactive change through feedback of results. In the UK, one NHS Trust found it reduced infection rates by about a third [11].

Antibiotic prophylaxis is a well-established method for minimizing the risk of SSI, although it is sometimes used inappropriately. In 2011, the English National Point Prevalence Survey on Healthcare-associated Infections and Antimicrobial Use showed that 13% of patients were on an antimicrobial for surgical prophylaxis, and of these 30% were administered for longer than 24 hours [12].

In this chapter we discuss optimization of this prophylaxis and provide examples of successful quality improvement programmes (QIPs) that have overcome the challenges.

Common principles of antibiotic prophylaxis

Prophylactic administration of antibiotics inhibits the growth of contaminating bacteria and their adherence to prosthetic implants, thus reducing the risk of infection:

The goals of prophylactic administration of antibiotics to surgical patients are to:

◆ Reduce the incidence of SSI

- Use antibiotics in a manner that is supported by evidence of effectiveness
- Minimise the effect of antibiotics on the patient's normal microbial flora
- Minimise adverse effects
- Cause minimal change to the patient's host defenses [13].

However, there are risks associated with prophylaxis and there is a delicate balance between reducing the risk of SSI and reducing the risk of adverse effects of antibiotics:

The final decision regarding the benefits and risks of prophylaxis for an individual patient will depend on:

- Patient's risk of SSI
- Potential severity of the consequences of SSI
- Effectiveness of prophylaxis for the procedure
- Consequences of prophylaxis for that patient e.g. increased risk of *Clostridium difficile* infection (CDI) [13].

Adverse events association with prophylaxis

Prophylaxis has the potential to cause many different adverse effects:

- allergy, the most serious manifestation being anaphylaxis
- side effects
- drug interactions
- effects on the patient's normal flora, possibly resulting in antibiotic-associated diarrhoea (including *Clostridium difficile* infection) or thrush
- development of resistance in the individual and the development and spread of resistance in the wider community.

Optimizing prophylaxis

The 'right drug, right dose, right time, right duration, right patient' mantra should be adopted (Table 13.1).

Local antibiotic stewardship teams have the experience and knowledge required to write specific guidelines based on an assessment of evidence, local information about resistance, and drug costs. However, guidelines should be written in conjunction with surgeons to encourage ownership of the guidance within the surgical team and thus improve compliance. It is also helpful to include anaesthetists in the creation and dissemination of the guidelines as they usually administer the antibiotic and may be responsible for prescribing.

Non-systemic antimicrobials may also be used to reduce SSI. Examples of this include topical decolonization of *Staphylococcus aureus*, antibiotic-impregnated bone cement and collagen sponges, and eye drops in ophthalmological surgery.

Quality improvement programmes and aids to prescribing

Examples of national quality improvement programmes

The Scottish Antimicrobial Prescribing Group (SAPG) have a well-established QIP that has successfully developed and embedded clinical antimicrobial management teams (AMTs) within

Table 13.1 Principles of surgical prophylaxis

Right drug	The antibiotic used must: ◆ be active against the most likely contaminating pathogens ◆ be the safest option available ◆ be the most cost-effective option available ◆ take into account local resistance patterns and trends as well as the patient's own colonizing flora, e.g. meticillin-resistant *Staphylococcus aureus* (MRSA) ◆ be the narrowest spectrum required to reduce impact on microbial flora and local resistance ◆ avoid cephalosporins, clindamycin, quinolones, and co-amoxiclav whenever possible to reduce the risks of *Clostridium difficile* infection (CDI) ◆ use appropriate alternatives for patients with penicillin/β-lactam allergy ◆ usually be given intravenously as absorption rates cannot be guaranteed following oral administration
Right dose	This is generally the same as the therapeutic dose and should provide adequate serum and tissue levels during the period of contamination. Dose adjustments may be required for: ◆ age ◆ body mass index or weight ◆ renal and liver function
Right time	The dose should be administered within the 60 minutes *prior* to surgical incision or tourniquet inflation to enable blood levels to exceed the minimum inhibitory concentration (MIC) of the target contaminating organisms from the start of the surgical procedure and throughout its duration. However, administration may be required to start up to 90–120 minutes prior to incision in the case of agents that have long infusion times, such as vancomycin
Right duration	Prophylaxis should be administered for the shortest effective period to minimize costs and risks: ◆ a single dose is effective in most cases ◆ up to 24 hours of prophylaxis may be warranted for certain procedures (e.g. primary arthroplasty) and for up to 48 hours for open heart surgery ◆ a repeat dose may be required for procedures lasting longer than the half-life of the antibiotic administered or for major intra-operative blood loss (>1500 ml in adults), in which case an additional dose should be considered after fluid replacement ◆ a treatment course of antibiotics may also need to be given (in addition to appropriate prophylaxis) in cases of dirty surgery or infected wounds
Right patient	Antimicrobial prophylaxis should be considered for surgical procedures associated with a high rate of infection and in some clean procedures where the consequences of infection are severe (e.g. prosthetic implants), even if infection is highly unlikely. Antibiotic prophylaxis should be given before: ◆ clean surgery involving the placement of a prosthesis or implant ◆ clean–contaminated surgery ◆ contaminated surgery Antibiotic prophylaxis should not be given routinely for clean, non-prosthetic uncomplicated surgery

Source: data from Scottish Intercollegiate Guidelines Network (SIGN), *Antibiotic prophylaxis in surgery*, SIGN publication no. 104, Edinburgh, UK, Copyright © 2008 SIGN; and Mertz et al., 'Does duration of perioperative antibiotic prophylaxis matter in cardiac surgery? A systematic review and meta-analysis,' *Annals of Surgery*, Volume 254, Issue 1, pp. 48–54, Copyright © 2011 Lippincott Williams.

NHS boards. These specialist teams are the key support for clinicians in primary and secondary care to encourage prudent prescribing. The formation of a clinical network of AMTs has been instrumental in providing SAPG with 'real world' feedback relating to antimicrobial issues. Their primary objective is to coordinate and deliver a national framework for antimicrobial stewardship to enhance the quality of antimicrobial prescribing and management. It strongly endorses adherence to the Scottish Intercollegiate Guideline Network (SIGN) guidelines, and one of its current quality improvement areas is surgical prophylaxis [14], the target indicator being 'duration of surgical antibiotic prophylaxis is <24 hours and compliant with local Antimicrobial Prescribing Policy' (target ≥95%) [15]. Surgical prophylaxis data were collected from 8 of 14 NHS boards for elective procedures in colorectal surgery (approximately 5600 elective procedures between April 2011 and June 2014). A case was 'compliant' if a given single dose of surgical antibiotic prophylaxis complied with the local surgical antibiotic prophylaxis policy: 98% received a single dose of antibiotics, and antibiotic choice complied with local policy in 92% of cases.

In 2003 the Surgical Care Improvement Project (SCIP) was created in North America. This is a national quality partnership of organizations committed to improving the safety of surgical care through the reduction of post-operative complications by developing a set of compliance measures [16–18]:

♦ SCIP-Inf-1: patients who received prophylactic antibiotics within 1 hour prior to surgical incision (2 hours if receiving vancomycin)

♦ SCIP-Inf-2: patients who received prophylactic antibiotics recommended for their specific surgical procedure

♦ SCIP-Inf-3: patients whose prophylactic antibiotics were discontinued within 24 hours after the end of surgery (48 hours for coronary artery bypass graft surgery or other cardiac surgery).

Cataife et al. [19] demonstrated that hospital groups with higher compliance rates had significantly lower SSI rates for two SCIP measures: antibiotic timing and appropriate antibiotic selection. For a hospital group with median characteristics, a 10% improvement in the measure 'provision of antibiotic 1 hour before intervention' led to a 5.3% decrease in SSI rates ($P < 0.05$). The analysis supports a clinically and statistically meaningful relationship between adherence to two SCIP measures and SSI rates, supporting the validity of the two publicly available HCAI metrics.

Examples of specific or local QIPs

At the Royal Devon and Exeter NHS Foundation Trust a monthly league table, 'The Champions League', was used to provide timely feedback on adherence to the Trust's surgical prophylaxis policy. The audit was performed by pharmacists and was displayed publicly each month. At the beginning, 53.5% of antibiotic courses had an indication documented and 53.5% had a review/stop date documented. Six months later, after two published league tables, 94.7% of antibiotic courses had the indication documented and 84.2% had the review/stop date documented. The use of one simple intervention led to a great improvement in prescribing habits [20].

Conclusion

Surgical prophylaxis reduces the risk of SSI-associated morbidity and mortality and associated costs in certain surgical and patient groups. However, the principles for prescribing surgical prophylaxis must be followed to reduce the risks of adverse events. To overcome the barriers to successful stewardship in this key area, organizations must have adequate surgical prophylaxis guidelines and policies, incorporating e-prescribing and new technologies, robust surveillance of SSIs, frequent audit with timely and effective feedback, and regular awareness and education programmes.

Acknowledgments

Text extracts from SIGN, *Antibiotic prophylaxis in surgery: A national clinical guideline*, reproduced by kind permission of the Scottish Intercollegiate Guidelines Network. Scottish Intercollegiate Guidelines Network (SIGN). *Antibiotic prophylaxis in surgery: A national clinical guideline*. Edinburgh: SIGN; 2008 and 2014. (SIGN publication no. 104). [16 June 2016]. Available from URL: http://www.sign.ac.uk

References

1 Smyth ET, McIlvenny G, Enstone JE, Emmerson AM, Humphreys H, Fitzpatrick F, et al. Four country healthcare associated infection prevalence survey 2006: overview of the results. *J Hosp Infect* 2008;**69**:230–48.

2 Astagneau P, Rioux C, Golliot F, Brucker G. Morbidity and mortality associated with surgical site infections: results from the 1997–1999 INCISO surveillance. *J Hosp Infect* 2001;**48**:267–74.

3 Zmistowski B, Karam JA, Durinka JB, Casper DS, Parvizi J. Periprosthetic joint infection increases the risk of one-year mortality. *J Bone Joint Surg Am* 2013;**95**:2177–84.

4 Coello R, Charlett A, Wilson J, Ward V, Pearson A, Borriello P. Adverse impact of surgical site infections in English hospitals. *J Hosp Infect* 2005;**60**:93–103.

5 Plowman R, Graves N, Griffin MA, Roberts JA, Swan AV, Cookson B, et al. The rate and cost of hospital-acquired infections occurring in patients admitted to selected specialties of a district general hospital in England and the national burden imposed. *J Hosp Infect* 2001;**47**:198–209.

6 Briggs TW. *Getting it right first time*. 2013. Available at: http://www.gettingitrightfirsttime.com/report/ (accessed 22 September 2014).

7 Johnson R, Jameson SS, Sanders RD, Sargant NJ, Muller SD, Meek RM, et al. Reducing surgical site infection in arthroplasty of the lower limb: a multi-disciplinary approach. *Bone Joint Res* 2013;**2**:58–65.

8 Dalfino L, Giglio MT, Puntillo F, Marucci M, Brienza N. Haemodynamic goal-directed therapy and postoperative infections: earlier is better. A systematic review and meta-analysis. *Crit Care* 2011;**15**:R154.

9 Newman JB, Bullock M, Goyal R. Comparison of glove donning techniques for the likelihood of gown contamination. An infection control study. *Acta Orthop Belg* 2007;**73**:765–71.

10 Wilson AP, Hodgson B, Liu M, Plummer D, Taylor I, Roberts J, et al. Reduction in wound infection rates by wound surveillance with postdischarge follow-up and feedback. *Br J Surg* 2006;**93**:630–8.

11 Plymouth Hospitals NHS Trust. Infection control win national patient safety award 2011. 2011. Available at: http://www.plymouthhospitals.nhs.uk/ourorganisation/newsandpublications/pressreleases/Pages/InfectionControlWinNationalPatientSafetyAward2011.aspx

12 Health Protection Agency. *English National Point Prevalence Survey on Healthcare Associated Infections and Antimicrobial Use, 2011: preliminary data*, 2012 London: Health Protection Agency.

13 Scottish Intercollegiate Guidelines Network. *Antibiotic prophylaxis in surgery*. Guideline **104**. 2014. Available at: http://sign.ac.uk/guidelines/fulltext/104/index.html

14 Scottish Medicines Consortium. Quality improvement. 2014. Available at: http://www.scottishmedicines.org.uk/SAPG/Quality_Improvement/Quality_Improvement (accessed 26 March 2015).

15 Scottish Antimicrobial Prescribing Group. Surgical prophylaxis indicator. AMT National Level Report April 2011–June 2014. 2014. Available from: https://www.scottishmedicines.org.uk/files/sapg1/Surgical_Prophylaxis_April_2011-_June_2014.pdf (accessed 15 May 2015).

16 **Bratzler DW, Hunt DR.** The surgical infection prevention and surgical care improvement projects: national initiatives to improve outcomes for patients having surgery. *Clin Infect Dis* 2006;**43**:322–30.

17 **Bratzler DW, Houck PM, Richards C, Steele L, Dellinger EP, Fry DE, et al.** Use of antimicrobial prophylaxis for major surgery: baseline results from the National Surgical Infection Prevention Project. *Arch Surg* 2005;**140**:174–82.

18 **Clancy CM.** SCIP: making complications of surgery the exception rather than the rule. *AORN J* 2008;**87**:621–4.

19 **Cataife G, Weinberg DA, Wong HH, Kahn KL.** The effect of Surgical Care Improvement Project (SCIP) compliance on surgical site infections (SSI). *Med Care* 2014;**52**(2 Suppl. 1):S66–S73.

20 **Evans JS, C. Armstrong, A.** The champions league—improving the quality of in-patient antibiotic prescription in trauma and orthopaedics. *BMJ Qual Improv Report* 2014;**3**.

Chapter 14

Antimicrobial stewardship in paediatrics

Sanjay Patel and Julia Bielicki

Introduction to antimicrobial stewardship in paediatrics

The paediatric perspective, that children are not just small adults, holds true for antimicrobial stewardship. Children pose unique challenges in terms of the aetiology of their infections, the non-specific nature of their infective presentations, the difficulty in obtaining adequate microbiological specimens, and the relative paucity of evidence on which to base decisions about treatment regimens in terms of choice of antimicrobial, dose, and duration.

The aetiology of infection in children

The majority of infective presentations to primary care physicians are for cough, coryzal symptoms, earache, sore throat, and gastroenteritis. Although the aetiology of these pathologies is often not accurately known, numerous pragmatic trials have shown that the administration of antibiotics makes little or no difference to the speed at which symptoms resolve [1,2]. In addition, the introduction of novel conjugate vaccines to the UK immunization schedule (Hib in 1992, meningococcal C in 1999, pneumococcal 7-valent in 2006, and pneumococcal 13-valent in 2010) has resulted in a marked reduction in the rate of invasive bacterial infection in children [3].

The selection of empiric regimens is based on the need to provide sufficient coverage. Children without chronic co-morbidities would not be expected to be colonized with resistant organisms such as meticillin-resistant *Staphylococcus aureus* (MRSA), vancomycin-resistant enterococcus (VRE), or carbapenem-resistant *Enterobacteriaceae* (CRE). However, in many cases the colonization status of hospitalized children is unknown. Resistance patterns of invasive isolates differ between children and adults, and the implications of this for empiric treatment are at present unclear, adding to the challenges of optimizing antibiotic treatment in this patient group.

Overall, therefore, making decisions about whether to commence and stop antibiotics in children is often challenging (see Box 14.1).

Patterns of prescribing in children

Antibiotic prescribing patterns for children differ markedly between primary and secondary care. While in the former setting antibiotics are overwhelmingly used for minor infections, inpatient antibiotic prescribing disproportionately targets children with often multiple and complex co-morbidities.

Box 14.1 Challenges in paediatric antibiotic prescribing—access to timely antibiotic therapy versus excessive use

- Severe childhood infection often presents with non-specific symptoms and signs, especially in infants and neonates
- Young infants (<3 months of age) are at considerably higher risk of invasive infection due to early and late-onset sepsis
- Commonly used point of care/rapid tests such as C-reactive protein may lack sensitivity in young children [4]
- Confirming a microbiological diagnosis is often difficult. Obtaining adequate blood volumes can be challenging and young children are unable to expectorate sputum

Source: data from Van den Bruel A et al. 2011 [4].

Primary care

Over the past 20 years, numerous national strategies have been implemented in an attempt to reduce the rate of antibiotic prescribing in primary care. Nevertheless, prescribing rates for common self-limiting pathologies such as sore throat, cough, and otitis media remain unchanged at about 50–60%, with marked variation between prescribers [5]. One of the challenges for prescribers is to distinguish between viral and bacterial infections. Clinicians are concerned that failure to treat a bacterial infection will result in severe infection or suppurative complications. However, data suggest that hundreds of patients need to be treated with antibiotics to avoid one serious complication following tonsillitis, otitis media, or an upper respiratory tract infection [6].

Secondary care

The Antibiotic Resistance and Prescribing in European Children (ARPEC) project provides the largest dataset on antibiotic prescribing in hospitalized children [7]. Subgroup analysis of UK hospitals showed that approximately 20% of children admitted to secondary care facilities are commenced on antibiotics, compared with 30% in tertiary centres. Along with children admitted to the paediatric intensive care unit (PICU) and haemato-oncology units, children with co-morbidities are most likely to be receiving antibiotics. Third-generation cephalosporins and broad-spectrum penicillins (amoxicillin/clavulanate) are the most commonly prescribed antibiotics, with low levels of carbapenems being prescribed. The most common indications for antibiotic prescribing are lower respiratory tract infections, followed by medical prophylaxis. Variability in prescribing rates between hospitals is striking and unlikely to be explained by differences in case mix alone [8].

Challenges in changing paediatric antimicrobial prescribing

In addition to the diagnostic challenges, there is a paucity of high-quality evidence on which to base decisions about antimicrobial prescribing in children in terms of the choice of empiric antibiotic, use of combination therapy, the total duration of treatment, and the timing of the intravenous to oral switch. This goes some way to explaining the large variability in prescribing habits between paediatric practitioners when treating a presumed bacterial infection.

Special populations

Children with underlying co-morbidities

Children with underlying co-morbidities, for example haemato-oncology patients or children with cystic fibrosis, can present unique challenges in terms of antimicrobial stewardship:

◆ These children are often vulnerable hosts in terms of impaired immunity and indwelling intravenous catheters. For this reason, empiric antimicrobial prescribing is likely to reflect a broader range of pathologies and pathogens. In addition, the potential for rapid deterioration often results in a lower threshold for commencing antibiotics.

◆ Approaches to antibiotic prescribing may be dictated by regional or national protocols.

◆ Children with co-morbidities are more likely to be colonized with resistant microorganisms. This often results in empiric treatment with broader-spectrum antibiotics.

Neonatal intensive care

The provision of neonatal intensive care has improved the survival of extremely premature and low-birthweight babies. However, prolonged neonatal intensive care unit (NICU) admission coupled with the relative immunodeficiency of premature neonates is associated with a high risk of invasive bacterial infection. Unsurprisingly therefore, NICU patients receive antibiotics at a much higher rate than the rate of confirmed infections. Exposure to broad-spectrum antibiotics has been found to be a risk factor for necrotizing enterocolitis and invasive candidaemia.

Hospital-acquired infections

Importantly, a European point prevalence survey of hospital-acquired infections (HAIs) found that bloodstream infections account for a particularly high proportion of paediatric HAIs compared with all other medical specialities, including intensive care [9]. This is likely to drive prescribing of broader-spectrum agents, and underlines the importance of clear, locally valid, and tailored empiric treatment recommendations as well as the key role of infection control as part of optimal paediatric antibiotic management [10].

Practical challenges in optimizing antibiotic management

The key personnel required to implement a successful hospital paediatric antimicrobial stewardship programme (PASP) include a paediatric infectious diseases consultant, a medical microbiologist, and a clinical pharmacist. In addition, close alignment with an infection prevention service is desirable. Unlike tertiary hospitals, most local hospitals are unlikely to have all of the listed key personnel.

There are also practical challenges in prescribing oral antibiotics for children. The choice of oral antibiotic should account for factors that can potentially affect adherence such as dosing frequency and the highly variable palatability/taste of formulations. Palatable oral drugs in a sensible regimen (up to three times a day) should be used whenever possible. Issues such as the need for dosing in the middle of the night to achieve optimal antibiotic pharmacokinetic/pharmacodynamic targets must be weighed against regimens that will maximize adherence.

Potential impact of a paediatric antimicrobial stewardship programme

As with studies conducted in adult patient populations, there is considerable evidence to support the introduction of PASPs (see Box 14.2).

Box 14.2 Impact of paediatric antimicrobial stewardship programmes

- Early detection of antimicrobial prescription errors [11]
- Reduced antimicrobial use and reduction in the evolution of resistance [12]
- Reduction in broad-spectrum antibiotic use [13]
- Significant cost savings [13]
- Positive impact on prescribing behaviour of clinicians

Source: data from Di Pentima MC et al. 2009 [10]; Di Pentima MC et al. 2011 [11]; and Metjian TA et al. 2008 [12].

One of the main challenges in paediatrics is to quantify the impact of a PASP on antibiotic prescribing. The most commonly used measure of adult prescribing is change in total defined daily dose (DDD; the assumed average maintenance dose per day for a drug used for its main indication in adults). Weight-based antibiotic dosing in children makes the interpretation of change in total DDD difficult and virtually precludes comparisons between hospitals for benchmarking. At present there is no standardized measure of antibiotic prescribing in children.

Strategies for successful implementation of a paediatric antimicrobial stewardship programme

If a PASP is to be successfully introduced, funding to employ the key personnel required for service delivery and buy-in from paediatric clinicians is essential.

Obtaining funding

- The potential impact of the planned PASP in terms of process measures (reduction in antibiotic prescribing), outcome measures (improved patient outcomes and reduced resistance), and economic measures (cost saving) must be demonstrated to hospital management.
- Focusing on high-use antibiotics in hospitals, such as third-generation cephalosporins, and common pathologies in the community, such as respiratory tract infections, is likely to have a far greater impact on antimicrobial prescribing than focusing on antibiotics that are currently rarely used, such as carbapenems.
- Harnessing existing structures for antimicrobial stewardship, such as an 'adult' medical microbiologist with additional specialist paediatric input, may enable hospitals to reduce costs by making use of efficiencies of scale.

Achieving buy-in from paediatric clinicians

- The identification of 'low-hanging fruit' is key—early successes are likely to result in early engagement from colleagues and management.
- Be seen to be promoting facilitation of improved antibiotic prescribing rather than restricting overall prescribing. Engaging in activities to improve processes such as the time taken to administer antibiotics in children with febrile neutropenia is likely to result in a better understanding that certain restrictive activities have the same purpose.

+ Identify local champions within various clinical areas. They can help bridge the gap between the PASP team and their colleagues.
+ Feeding back data that demonstrate the impact of PASP interventions is likely to achieve continued buy-in from clinicians.

Children—the take home message

Promoting and monitoring the judicious use of antimicrobials in children poses unique challenges. Confirming a microbiological diagnosis can be difficult, and there is often a paucity of evidence informing decision making about antimicrobial prescribing. In addition, there is currently no standardized measure of antibiotic prescribing in children. Different antimicrobial stewardship strategies tailored to neonates and children are required in primary and secondary/tertiary care settings.

References

1 Venekamp RP, Sanders S, Glasziou PP, Del Mar CB, Rovers MM. Antibiotics for acute otitis media in children. *Cochrane Database Syst Rev* 2013;(1):CD000219.

2 Spinks A, Glasziou PP, Del Mar CB. Antibiotics for sore throat. *Cochrane Database Syst Rev* 2013;(11):CD000023.

3 Le Doare K, Nichols AL, Payne H, Wells R, Navidnia S, Appleby G, et al. Very low rates of culture-confirmed invasive bacterial infections in a prospective 3-year population-based surveillance in southwest London. *Arch Dis Child* 2014;**99**:526–31.

4 Van den Bruel A, Thompson MJ, Haj-Hassan T, Stevens R, Moll H, Lakhanpaul M, et al. Diagnostic value of laboratory tests in identifying serious infections in febrile children: systematic review. *Br Med J* 2011;**342**:d3082.

5 Hawker JI, Smith S, Smith GE, Morbey R, Johnson AP, Fleming DM, et al. Trends in antibiotic prescribing in primary care for clinical syndromes subject to national recommendations to reduce antibiotic resistance, UK 1995–2011: analysis of a large database of primary care consultations. *J Antimicrob Chemother* 2014;**69**:3423–30.

6 Petersen I, Johnson AM, Islam A, Duckworth G, Livermore DM, Hayward AC. Protective effect of antibiotics against serious complications of common respiratory tract infections: retrospective cohort study with the UK General Practice Research Database. *Br Med J* 2007;**335**:982.

7 Versporten A, Sharland M, Bielicki J, Drapier N, Vankerckhoven V, Goossens H. The antibiotic resistance and prescribing in European Children project: a neonatal and pediatric antimicrobial web-based point prevalence survey in 73 hospitals worldwide. *Pediatr Infect Dis J* 2013;**32**:e242–e253.

8 Katja Doerholt, St Georges Hospital, London, personal communication.

9 European Centre for Disease Prevention and Control. *ECDC surveillance report. Point prevalence survey of healthcare-associated infections and antimicrobial use in European acute care hospitals 2011–2012.* Available at: http://ecdc.europa.eu/en/publications/Publications/healthcare-associated-infections-antimicrobial-use-PPS.pdf

10 Posfay-Barbe KM, Zerr DM, Pittet D. Infection control in paediatrics. *Lancet Infect Dis* 2008;**8**:19–31.

11 Di Pentima MC, Chan S, Eppes SC, Klein JD. Antimicrobial prescription errors in hospitalized children: role of antimicrobial stewardship program in detection and intervention. *Clin Pediatr* 2009;**48**:505–12.

12 Di Pentima MC, Chan S, Hossain J. Benefits of a pediatric antimicrobial stewardship program at a children's hospital. *Pediatrics* 2011;**128**:1062–70.

13 Metjian TA, Prasad PA, Kogon A, Coffin SE, Zaoutis TE. Evaluation of an antimicrobial stewardship program at a pediatric teaching hospital. *Pediatr Infect Dis J* 2008;**27**:106–11.

Chapter 15

Stewardship in the primary care and long-term care settings

Naomi Fleming

Introduction to stewardship in the primary care and long-term care settings

Antibiotic prescribing in the community accounts for 80% of all antibiotic prescribing; approximately 75% of this is for acute respiratory tract infections (RTIs), many of which are viral [1]. The majority of this prescribing is in primary care; however, other settings include urgent care, community health services, community-based outpatient parenteral antibiotic therapy (OPAT) services, offender care settings, and long-term care facilities (LTCF).

Pharmacists are employed in many community settings, but there are few dedicated antimicrobial pharmacists in the community, with stewardship being an addition to rather than the focus of their role. A survey of primary care trusts (PCTs) showed that 23% (of the 108 which responded) had a substantive primary care antimicrobial prescribing adviser [2].

This chapter will focus on primary care and LTCF identifying stewardship activities and challenges within these settings along with practical examples.

Primary care

There is wide variation between general practices in antibiotic prescribing rates that cannot be explained by differences in the epidemiology of infections, populations, or case mix [3]. There is no single intervention that will be successful in all practices, and multifaceted interventions along with addressing local barriers to change are the most effective types. Their effectiveness is often dependent on the prescribing behaviours, experiences, and local challenges seen in a particular practice or an individual general practitioner (GP) [4,5]. The TARGET toolkit (for 'treat antibiotics responsibly, guidelines, education, tools'), takes a multifaceted approach and contains many antimicrobial stewardship (AMS) resources for use in primary care, including guidelines, audit tools, and patient information [6].

Components of AMS programmes

Guidelines

There is limited access to microbiological laboratories in primary care, therefore initial prescribing is empiric. The majority of organisms causing infections in the community are predictable, for example *Escherichia coli* urinary tract infections (UTIs). National empiric guidelines targeting these organisms are issued by Public Health England (PHE) for use in the primary care setting [7]. These guidelines are updated regularly with changes in resistance patterns and new evidence. They encourage prescribers to use narrow-spectrum antibiotics and describe key components of AMS. A survey showed 90 out of 108 responding PCTs used these guidelines to develop their local guidance [2]. There are also national and locally developed condition-specific guidelines with details on diagnostic criteria and factors that may influence antibiotic choice, for example National Institute for Health and Care Excellence (NICE) guidelines on the diagnosis of community-acquired and hospital-acquired pneumonia (CAP and HAP, respectively) [8].

Educational strategies

Educational strategies including lectures, meetings at practices, written materials, and e-learning packages have shown varied success. The Stemming the Tide of Antibiotic Resistance (STAR) educational programme included a practice-based seminar reflecting on the practice's own dispensing and resistance data, online educational elements, and practising consulting skills in routine care; it was found that its use in GP practices led to a 4.2% reduction in total oral antibiotic dispensing, with no significant change in admissions to hospital, re-consultations, or costs [3].

Delayed prescribing

A prescription is written by the GP but the patient is encouraged only to fulfil it if they are not better within a set time frame or have deteriorated. The prescription may be given to the patient at the initial consultation with advice, or may be kept at the surgery so that the patient has to collect it before getting it dispensed. The NICE clinical guideline 'Respiratory tract infections—antibiotic prescribing: prescribing of antibiotics for self-limiting respiratory tract infections in adults and children in primary care' [9] advocates the use of a delayed prescribing strategy. Studies on sore throat have shown that if the collection of the prescription is delayed for 72 hours, collection is reduced by 69% and future consultations for sore throats also fall [10]. A Cochrane review [11] of delayed antibiotic prescribing in all acute RTIs, showed that delayed prescribing significantly reduced antibiotic use compared with immediate prescribing (32% versus 93%), but a no-prescribing strategy resulted in the least antibiotic use (14%). Patient satisfaction was slightly reduced in the delayed group, similar to the no-antibiotic group. Clinical outcomes, adverse effects, complications, and re-consultation rates showed little difference. The authors concluded that in patients with RTIs for whom clinicians feel it is safe not to prescribe antibiotics immediately, no antibiotics with advice to return if symptoms do not resolve is likely to result in the least antibiotic use, while maintaining similar patient satisfaction and clinical outcomes to delayed antibiotics.

Point of care testing

Laboratory results such as white cell counts and C-reactive protein (CRP) are not currently routinely available in primary care at consultation. A study by Cals et al. [12] showed that a combination of communication skills training and CRP point of care testing in lower RTIs safely reduced antibiotic prescribing without reducing satisfaction with care. Point of care CRP testing is recommended in NICE clinical guideline 191 [8] for people presenting to primary care with a lower RTI if a diagnosis of pneumonia has not been made and it is not clear whether antibiotics should be prescribed. Immediate, delayed, or no prescribing strategies for antibiotics are guided by the result.

Audit and feedback

Practice can be compared with guidelines to show how practice is inconsistent with a target, for example a target for cephalosporin prescribing, or to compare practices or prescribers, for example peer comparisons of prescribing data. Antimicrobial consumption data are often used, although condition-specific audits can be undertaken, for example the sore throat audit tool from TARGET [6]. A Cochrane review of the effects on professional practice and healthcare outcomes across all types of prescribing and behaviours [13] showed that this approach leads to small but potentially important improvements.

Quality improvement targets

Quality improvement initiatives such as quality outcome frameworks (QOF), quality, innovation, productivity, and prevention (QIPP) comparators, and local prescribing incentive schemes can be used to influence antibiotic prescribing. QOF rewards practices for the provision of quality care. QIPP comparators aim to support prescribers to review the appropriateness of current prescribing, revise prescribing, and monitor implementation. They highlight variation and support local decisions regarding QIPP and local prescribing incentive schemes [14].

National QIPP comparators include the following:

- 3 days trimethoprim average daily quantity (ADQ)/item
- minocycline ADQ/1000 patients
- antibacterial items/STAR PU (specific therapeutic group age–sex weightings-related prescribing units)
- cephalosporins—per cent of total antibiotic items
- quinolones—per cent of total antibiotic items
- co-amoxiclav, cephalosporins, and quinolones—combined per cent of total antibiotic items

Nationally, cephalosporin prescribing in primary care has approximately halved and quinolone prescribing has reduced by around 38% across England since April 2007 (see Box 15.1) [15].

Patient-targeted interventions

Patent-targeted interventions include shared decision making, provision of written information, public education events, and national campaigns such as the antibiotic guardian campaign, part of the 2014 European Antibiotics Awareness Day. The EQUIP study [17] demonstrated that an in-consultation booklet completed with parents safely reduced antibiotic prescribing for children.

Box 15.1 Practical points

To address the variation in prescribing volume seen between Milton Keynes Clinical Commissioning Group (CCG) and national average antibiotic prescribing volumes, a mandatory QOF target was developed based on a locally adapted antimicrobial self-assessment toolkit [16]. It included sections on guidelines, education, delayed prescribing, audit, patient advice, and implementation of local feedback reports. This target ran from April 2012 to March 2014. The aim of the first year was to develop an action plan so that in second year the practice would achieve 18/20, i.e. 90%. The variation in antibiotic prescribing volume (MKCCG versus national) fell from 121 items per STAR-PU to 107 in the first year and to 67 in the second year, a reduction in variation of 47% (Figure 15.1).

A prescribing incentive scheme target for co-amoxiclav of <5% of total antibiotic prescribing over the same period reduced the CCG's average co-amoxiclav prescribing by 19% in the first year and a further 7% in the second year, compared with national prescribing which rose 3% in the first year and then fell 3% in the second year (Figure 15.2).

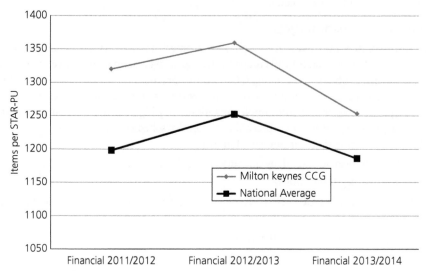

Figure 15.1 Antibiotics per STAR-PU Milton Keynes Clinical Commissioning Group average versus national average.

Source: data from ePACT.net.

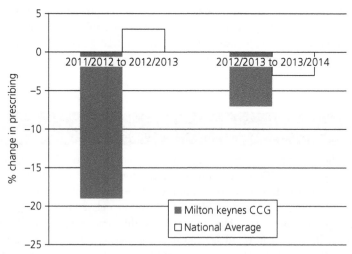

Figure 15.2 Reduction in co-amoxiclav prescribing (%)Milton Keynes Clinical Commissioning Group (MKCCG) average versus national average.

Source: data from ePACT.net.

Challenges

One of the main challenges for improving antibiotic prescribing is patient demand [18]. Patients who do not have knowledge about the harms of antibiotic prescribing and antibiotic resistance are more likely to demand antibiotics or re-consult at the practice or urgent care setting. Patients may also complain and leave the practice if they feel strongly, leading to a loss of business for the practice and potentially adversely affecting the NHS outcome framework measures on patient experience. Prescriber perception of patient demand is inaccurate. A study by Macfarlane et al. in 1997 [19] showed that prescribers overestimate patient demand. Patients actually want symptomatic relief and an explanation of their illness—a patient information leaflet (PIL) reduced re-consultation for further illness, whether or not an antibiotic was given [20].

There is a perceived increase in workload at the initial consultation if time is taken to explain why antibiotics are not being given and then a presumed re-consultation; however, the evidence shows that by educating patients and not prescribing antibiotics, re-consultation rates actually fall.

GPs have many targets and are reluctant to make any changes that may adversely affect these targets, some of which can be interpreted to compete with the AMS agenda—for example targets to reduce admissions to secondary care and consultations at urgent care services. Reducing premature mortality from respiratory disease and preventing lower RTIs in children from becoming serious are part of the NHS outcomes framework [21].

There are also important competing clinical issues such as care of the elderly, long-term conditions, and mental health, and it is difficult for one topic to retain the clinical focus of GPs.

GPs have limited access to diagnostic tools and prescribe antibiotics empirically in response to symptoms. There is concern about missing a bacterial infection that leads to a poor patient outcome or litigation. This, combined with the lack of seeing the adverse events, such as antibiotic resistance or *Clostridium difficile*, in the majority of their patients leads to GPs being overly cautious and prescribing antibiotics inappropriately.

Long-term care facilities

There are limited published data on AMS in LTCF with most evidence coming from overseas. A recent systematic review reported that 47–79% of nursing home residents in the USA received systemic antimicrobials each year [22]. Older people have a high incidence of infection due to underlying co-morbidities, the use of invasive devices, and lowered immunity; they are susceptible to infection due to transmission of infection within their environment and are frequently colonized with multiresistant organisms [23,24]. However, up to three-quarters of antibiotic prescriptions for residents are reported to be inappropriate [25]. Prescribing is initiated to mange symptoms, often reported on the telephone by staff [26], or for non-specific clinical alterations attributed to infection when evidence to confirm infection is not present [27,28].

AMS strategies

There are no standard approaches to AMS across LTCF, but several studies have been described in a recent review [24]. One report from the USA described an AMS team of an infectious diseases physician and a nurse practitioner who visited weekly and were available for telephone advice. Ninety-five per cent of their recommendations were followed and total antimicrobial use was reduced by 30%. There was also a reduction in positive *C. difficile* tests. One trial in Canada including eight LTCFs involved posting a prescribing guide and individual prescribing profile to physicians in the intervention group at initiation and at month four. There was significant improvement in antimicrobial prescribing reported for the intervention group during the 3 months following the second information delivery.

Some of the reports in the review concerned interventions targeted at specific infections; these had varied success, with the studies targeting pneumonia reporting no impact on antimicrobial use for this indication. Studies addressing UTIs were reported to be effective, showing a decrease in the number of days prescribed for a suspected UTI, reductions in the proportion of inappropriate urine specimens sent for culture, and a reduction in episodes of treatment of asymptomatic bacteriuria. A study to address widespread use of long-term prophylaxis for UTIs also reduced use from 13% in 2005 to 6% in 2008 [24].

Challenges

There is difficulty in assessing elderly patients who may not show the same symptoms as younger patients, and there is often diagnostic uncertainty due to a lack of microbiological testing.

GPs may prescribe without visiting the patient, relying on staff to relay information and symptoms. Staff who contact prescribers about their residents have a range of medical knowledge. Nursing homes employ nurses, but care homes employ staff with no medical qualifications, English may not be their first language, and personal beliefs may play a part in their decision making.

There is a desire to treat residents before they become seriously unwell and need admitting to hospital and there is pressure from the patient's family to do all that is possible for their relative.

Overview

AMS in LTCF is not well defined and is an area that needs development. Studies have shown that improvements in antimicrobial use can be achieved in this setting, but more research in the UK is necessary.

References

1 Gill JM, Fleichut P, Haas S, Pellini B, Crawford A, Nash DB. Use of antibiotics for adult upper respiratory infections in outpatient settings: a national ambulatory network study. *Fam Med* 2006;**38**:349–54.

2 McNulty CAM, Guise T, Hand K, Howard P, Dryden M Cooke J. Antimicrobial stewardship in primary care—what are pharmacists doing? *Pharmaceutical J* October 2012.

3 Butler CC, Simpson SA, Dunstan F, Rollnick S, Cohen D, Gillespie D, et al. Effectiveness of multifaceted educational programme to reduce antibiotic dispensing in primary care: practice based randomised controlled trial. *Br Med J* 2012;**344**:d8173.

4 Arnold SR, Straus SE. Interventions to improve antibiotic prescribing practices in ambulatory care. *Cochrane Database Syst Rev* 2005;(4):CD003539.

5 Harris DJ. Initiatives to improve appropriate antibiotic prescribing in primary care. *J Antimicrob Chemother* 2013;**68**:2424–7.

6 Royal College of General Practitioners. TARGET antibiotics toolkit. 2012. Available at: http://www.rcgp.org.uk/TARGETantibiotics (accessed 31 March 2015).

7 **Public Health England. Management of infection guidance for primary care for consultation and local adaptation.** November 2012, revised February 2013. https://www.gov.uk/government/publications/managing-common-infections-guidance-for-primary-care (last accessed 31 March 2015)

8 National Institute for Health and Care Excellence. Clinical guideline 191. Pneumonia in adults: diagnosis and management. 2014. Available at: http://www.nice.org.uk/guidance/cg191 (last accessed 31 March 2015).

9 National Institute for Health and Care Excellence. Respiratory tract infections (self-limiting): prescribing antibiotics. 2008 (reviewed 2014). http://guidance.nice.org.uk/CG69 (last accessed 31 March 2015).

10 Little P, Williamson I, Warner G, Gould C, Gantley M, Kinmonth AL, et al. Open randomised trial of prescribing strategies in managing sore throat. *Br Med J* 1997;**314**:722–7.

11 Spurling GKP, Del Mar CB, Dooley L, Foxlee R, Farley R. Delayed antibiotics for respiratory infections. *Cochrane Database Syst Rev* 2013;(4):CD004417.

12 Cals JW, Butler CC, Hopstaken RM, Hood K, Dinant GJ. Effect of point of care testing for C reactive protein and training in communication skills on antibiotic use in lower respiratory tract infections: cluster randomised trial. *Br Med J* 2009;**338**:b1374.

13 Ivers N, Jamtvedt G, Flottorp S, Young JM, Odgard-Jensen J, French SD, et al. Audit and feedback: effects on professional practice and healthcare outcomes. *Cochrane Database Syst Rev* 2012:(6):CD000259.

14 National Health Services Business Authority. QIPP prescribing comparators. 2013. Available at: http://www.nhsbsa.nhs.uk/PrescriptionServices/3332.aspx (accessed 31 March 2015).

15 National Health Services Business Authority. Antibiotics national charts. 2013. Available at: http://www.nhsbsa.nhs.uk/PrescriptionServices/Documents/PPDPrescribingAnalysisCharts/Antibiotics_Jun_2013_National.pdf (accessed 31 March 2015).

16 Cooke J, Alexander K, Charani E, Hand K, Hills T, Howard P, et al. Antimicrobial stewardship: an evidence-based, antimicrobial self-assessment toolkit (ASAT) for acute hospitals. *J Antimicrob Chemother* 2010;**65**:2669–73.

17 Francis NA, Butler CC, Hood K, Simpson S, Wood F, Nuttall J. Effect of using an interactive booklet about childhood respiratory tract infections in primary care consultations on reconsulting and antibiotic prescribing: a cluster randomised controlled trial. *Br Med J* 2009;**339**: b2885.

18 Akkerman AE, Kuyvenhoven MM, van der Wouden JC, Verheij TJ. Determinants of antibiotic overprescribing in respiratory tract infections in general practice. *J Antimicrob Chemother* 2005;**56**:930–6.

19 Macfarlane J, Holmes W, Macfarlane R, Britten N. Influence of patients' expectations on antibiotic management of acute lower respiratory tract illness in general practice: questionnaire study. *Br Med J* 1997;**315**:1211–14.

20 Macfarlane JT, Holmes W, Macfarlane R. Reducing reconsultations for acute lower respiratory tract illness with an information leaflet: a randomized controlled study of patients in primary care. *Br J Gen Pract* 1997;**47**:719–22.

21 National Health Services Commissioning Board. NHS outcomes framework and CCG outcomes indicators: data availability table. 2012. Available at: http://www.england.nhs.uk/wp-content/uploads/2012/12/oi-data-table.pdf (accessed 31 March 2015).

22 van Buul LW, van der Steen JT, Veenhuizen RB, Achterberg WP, Schellevis FG, Essink RTGM, et al. Antibiotic use and resistance in long term care facilities. *J Am Med Dir Assoc* 2012;**13**:568.e1–568.e13.

23 Friedman ND. Antimicrobial stewardship: the need to cover all bases. *Antibiotics* 2013;**2**:400–18.

24 Nicolle L. Antimicrobial stewardship in long term care facilities: what is effective? *Antimicrob Resist Infect Control* 2014;**3**:6

25 Nicolle LE, Bentley DW, Garibaldi R, Neuhaus EG, Smith PW. Antimicrobial use in long-term care facilities. *Infect Control Hosp Epidemiol* 2000;**21**:537–45.

26 Richards CLJr, Darradji M, Weinberg A, Ouslander JG. Antimicrobial use in post-acute care: a retrospective descriptive analysis in seven long-term care facilities in Georgia. *J Am Med Dir Assoc* 2005;**6**:109–12.

27 Stone ND, Ashraf MS, Calder J, Crinch CJ, Crossley K, Drinka PJ, et al. Surveillance definitions of infections in long-term care facilities: revisiting the McGeer criteria. *Infect Control Hosp Epidemiol* 2012;**33**:965–77.

28 McGeer A, Campbell B, Emori T, Hierholzer WJ, Jackson MM, Nicolle LE, et al. Definitions of infection for surveillance in long-term facilities. *Am J Infect Control* 1991;**19**:1–7.

Chapter 16

Antifungal stewardship

Laura Whitney and Tihana Bicanic

Introduction to antifungal stewardship

The aims of antifungal stewardship (AFS) are broadly similar to those of antibiotic stewardship, namely to reduce inappropriate use and improve patient outcomes while reducing the evolution and spread of microbial resistance. Nevertheless, there are several key differences (Table 16.1). It should also be noted that limiting the use of antibacterials through antibiotic stewardship also contributes to AFS by reducing one driver of *Candida* infections.

Background

Due to the rarity of invasive fungal infection (IFI) and the lower incidence of resistance relative to bacteria, AFS has received comparably less attention than antibiotic stewardship and thus has a more limited evidence base [1]. However, AFS is gaining momentum as increasing populations are placed at risk of IFI and healthcare services become more cost-conscious. Moreover, fungal resistance has been described in several contexts [2–5], with selection pressure driven by the over-use of antifungals playing a key role in its emergence, leading to ineffective treatment, morbidity and mortality, and excess healthcare costs [6–8]. Cost is a major driver for AFS as antifungals are

Table 16.1 Differences between antifungal and antibiotic stewardship

	Antibacterial stewardship	Antifungal stewardship
Setting	Primary and secondary care	Mainly secondary care
Specialities involved	All specialities	Fewer specialities: haemato-oncology, organ transplantation, critical care, gastrointestinal surgery, respiratory
Indication	Mainly treatment or single-dose prophylaxis	Prolonged prophylaxis and treatment
Availability and cost	Many drugs, cost £–££s	Fewer drugs, expensive ££–£££
Resistance	Increasing multidrug resistance	Mono-resistance: multidrug resistance only a clinical issue in *Candida glabrata* to date
Pharmacokinetics	Less complex—few interactions	Complex—many interactions and contraindications, therapeutic drug monitoring indicated (azoles)
UK funding stream	In tariff	Payment by results exempt

significantly more expensive than the most commonly used antibiotics (Figure 16.1), therefore an AFS programme can be highly cost-effective.

Several key issues contribute to the overuse of antifungals and must be addressed by AFS:

♦ Inadequate knowledge of prescribers about the management of IFI [9].

♦ Lack of (access to) rapid, sensitive, and specific fungal diagnostics to facilitate accurate and timely diagnosis, leading to excessive empiric prescribing.

♦ Vulnerability of high-risk patient groups with high mortality attributable to IFI [10–12], even with appropriate treatment, leading to reluctance to delay treatment.

♦ Difficult prescribing decisions due to the complexity of the evidence base supporting treatment and prophylaxis, the need for individualized pharmacist input regarding drug interactions, inter- and intrapatient variations in pharmacokinetics/pharmacodynamics (PK/PD), and the need for therapeutic drug monitoring (TDM).

These issues inform the aims of and strategies for AFS and are detailed in Box 16.1. Key elements that differ from antibacterial stewardship are discussed in the rest of this chapter.

Post-prescription review with de-escalation

Balancing the need to give prompt effective therapy where appropriate, while avoiding the use of an antifungal when not indicated, remains the most challenging aspect of AFS. Delays in appropriate treatment are associated with increased mortality [13], but diagnostic difficulties and delays mean that a large proportion of antifungal use is empiric [10–14]. Therefore improving access to accurate diagnostics and timely specialist clinical review play a large part in stewardship.

De-escalation can be challenging as invasive mould infection may be diagnosed histologically, radiologically, or using biomarkers, meaning that susceptibility results are not always available to guide therapy. Even when microbiological susceptibility is confirmed there may be scope to improve de-escalation; studies of patients with candidaemia have shown that fewer than 40% of echinocandin-treated patients with fluconazole-susceptible isolates were de-escalated [14,15].

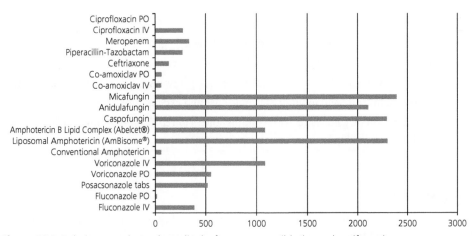

Figure 16.1 Relative costs (pounds sterling) of common antibiotics and antifungals.

Source: data from British Medical Association and the Royal Pharmaceutical Society, *BNF*, Copyright © BMJ Group and the Royal Pharmaceutical Society of Great Britain 2015, available from https://www.medicinescomplete.com/mc/bnf/current/index.htm (accessed March 2015).

Box 16.1 Aims and suggested components of an antifungal stewardship programme

Aims of AFS

- To optimize care of patients with IFI
- To stop unnecessary empiric treatment
- To de-escalate antifungal therapy when appropriate
- To ensure that TDM is performed when indicated and therapy is modified according to results
- To reduce antifungal usage and expenditure, without compromising on clinical outcome or resistance rates

Suggested components of an AFS programme

- Creation of a multidisciplinary AFS team (core members microbiology/infectious diseases specialist and a clinical pharmacist)
- Restriction of antifungals
- Post-prescription review with feedback including:
  - cessation of unnecessary treatment
  - de-escalation
  - intravenous to oral switch
  - optimizing non-drug treatment—source control, restoring immunity, or reducing immunosuppression
  - optimizing drug usage—ensuring appropriate dosing taking into account PK/PD, interactions, TDM, hepatic/renal dysfunction, and managing and preventing adverse drug reactions
- education
- Optimizing access to and turn-around time of fungal diagnostics
- Regular review of local fungal epidemiology including rates of resistance
- Implementation of evidence-based guidelines/care pathways, adapted to the local setting
- Processes to measure and monitor antifungal use and expenditure
- Implementation of 'gain share' with commissioners to recoup cost savings for individual NHS Trusts (in the UK)

Diagnostics

Restricting empiric antifungal use relies on improved diagnostics; therefore advances in biomarker-based and molecular diagnostics are likely to enhance AFS [1]. Studies show a reduction in antifungal use associated with the adoption of a diagnostic-driven approach incorporating non-culture-based tests, such as galactomannan and *Aspergillus* polymerase chain reaction (PCR), along with radiology [16–19]. Harnessing the excellent negative predictive value of these tests to exclude invasive aspergillosis and curtail empiric prescribing [20] is an AFS strategy that has been associated with savings in expenditure on antifungals without increasing mortality [17].

For candidaemia, recently developed rapid diagnostic techniques such as peptide nucleic acid fluorescence *in situ* hybridization (PNA-FISH), multiplex PCR, and matrix-assisted laser desorption/ionization time-of-flight mass spectrometry (MALDI-TOF-MS), can aid the stewardship process by improving the accuracy and timeliness (minutes to hours rather than 1–2 days) of identification of *Candida* species from positive blood cultures, allowing earlier tailoring of empiric therapy [21–23] (see Chapter 10).

Timely access to radiological investigations and bronchoscopy is also a key part of AFS, not only to optimize prescribing decisions and clinical review, but also because the diagnostic utility of such tests is time dependent, with the characteristic radiological features of invasive aspergillosis being transient [24]. The use of rapid diagnostics on bronchoalveolar lavage fluid in particular has been associated with improved inpatient outcomes [25].

In addition, optimizing diagnostics informs local antifungal guidelines through knowledge of local epidemiology.

Implementing an AFS programme—the evidence base

The published literature on AFS programmes is summarized in Table 16.2 [26–30]. Five key papers have been identified, detailing different stewardship strategies in different clinical settings.

At our own institution, data from the first 3 years (2010–13) of weekly AFS rounds have shown [31]:

- One-third of prescribing was empiric, of which the majority (82%) was unnecessary (just 3% of patients treated empirically had proven or probable infection)
- Significant sub-optimal management of IFIs and prophylactic prescribing (68% of reviews resulted in an intervention)
- Advice was well received by physicians (acceptance rate = 81%)
- Sustained reductions in antifungal consumption and expenditure can be achieved with limited resources (£100 000 year-on-year savings on drug acquisition costs, using 3 hours infectious diseases consultant and pharmacist time per week), rendering the programme highly cost-effective

Our programme has been successfully replicated in another large teaching hospital, which showed similar scope for interventions [32].

Implementing an AFS programme—keys to success

The initial goals of an AFS programme should be modest, allowing demonstration of success in the short term [1]. This can be achieved by targeting a few high-cost antifungal drugs, which are sub-optimally utilized, focusing on specialities with high antifungal usage (e.g. the intensive care unit or haematology) or using microbiological diagnosis to prompt clinical review (e.g. appropriate de-escalation in invasive candidiasis).

Assertive persuasion is an essential communication skill for members of the team when developing an AFS programme. Attention should be paid to reviewing literature on the prevention and management of IFIs, updating local antifungal guidelines, evaluating on-site diagnostic capacity and turn-around-time (microbiology, radiology, bronchoscopy), generating close working relationships with departments with high antifungal usage (to build confidence around advice acceptance, especially de-escalation), and ensuring accurate methods for identifying antifungal prescriptions for review.

Table 16.2 Summary of published reports of antifungal stewardship programmes

Study	Setting	AFS team	AFS intervention employed	Additional strategies in place prior to intervention	Primary objective	Outcome(s)
López-Medrano et al. (2013) [28]	1300-bed university hospital, Madrid, Spain	Infectious diseases and microbiology department	ID doctor spent 3 h every weekday reviewing all new AF prescriptions for L-amphotericin, caspofungin, and voriconazole, those eligible for modification and all patients with positive fungal cultures. Non-compulsory recommendations made verbally or in medical notes	Nil	Reduction in antifungal expenditure	Interventions made for 29% of 662 treatments reviewed: ◆ 15% IV–oral switch ◆ 8% stop ◆ 6% switch to fluconazole Advice acceptance 99% Reduced caspofungin and IV voriconazole use by 31% and 20% respectively Increased L-amphotericin and oral voriconazole use by 14% and 8% respectively Reduction in AF spend of 12%, saving US$370 682 over a 12-month period No significant change in local epidemiology
Apisarnthanarak et al (2010) [27]	350-bed tertiary care hospital, Bangkok, Thailand	Two ID specialists, one clinical microbiologist, four pharmacists, two internists, a hospital epidemiologist, an infection control specialist, and a computer systems analyst	Invasive candidiasis only. Successive introduction of: ◆ baseline audit of Candida species causing infection, AF prescribing and costs with feedback to prescribers ◆ AF order forms ◆ bedside case-management discussions by AFS team and attending physicians	Treatment and prophylaxis guidelines	To evaluate changes in AF prescribing, azole consumption, and incidence of infections caused by Candida albicans versus non-albicans species, and to estimate costs associated with the implementation of the AFS programme	59% reduction in AF prescriptions Significant reduction in the frequency of azole prescriptions compared with pre-intervention period (251 versus 124 DDDs per 1000 patient-days) Significant reduction in fluconazole use (from 242 to 117 DDDs per 1000 patient-days) Cost savings in AF use of US$31 615 over 1.5 years Reduced incidence of C. glabrata and C. krusei infections with increased incidence of C. albicans infection associated with changes in fluconazole use

Study	Setting	Team	Intervention	Study aim	Results
			◆ educational tool for hepatic/renal dose adjustments ◆ AF prescription forms ◆ monthly educational meetings ◆ restriction of polyene, azole, and echinocandin drugs		Appropriate AF use increased from 24% to 71% No difference in crude mortality
Reed et al. (2014) [30]	1229-bed teaching hospital, Ohio, USA	ID physicians, pharmacists, and microbiologists	Pharmacist notification by microbiology (during 'office hours') when yeast consistent with *Candida* spp. identified on Gram stain from a positive blood culture Pharmacist reviewed patient and recommended: ◆ AF therapy if not already initiated ◆ ID and ophthalmology consults ◆ CVC removal, when appropriate ◆ de-escalation and IV-PO switch once appropriate Guidelines for pharmacological management of candidaemia Notification of positive *Candida* blood culture to physician/nurse 24 h/day, 7 days/week	Evaluation of time to effective antifungal therapy before and after AFS programme	Significantly shorter median time from Gram stain result to effective AF therapy during 'office hours' (1.3 versus 13.5 h) Significantly more patients (99% versus 88%) received effective AF therapy A trend towards longer durations of effective therapy, higher number of ID consults, and more echocardiograms obtained Significantly more ophthalmology consults Significantly more patients received fluconazole PO as a result of pharmacist interventions (35% versus 21%) No significant change in LOS, infection-related LOS, total hospital costs, hospital costs during candidaemia, or in-hospital mortality No significant difference in *Candida* spp. isolated pre- and post-intervention in both study periods

(continued)

Table 16.2 Continued

Study	Setting	AFS team	AFS intervention employed	Additional strategies in place prior to intervention	Primary objective	Outcome(s)
Alfandari et al. (2014) [26]	Regional teaching hospital, Lille, France	ID specialists, haematologists	Twice weekly visits by ID specialist to haematology unit to discuss all patients with suspected infection. In non-haematology settings patients were reviewed at the physician's request	Treatment and prophylaxis guidelines	Not described	40% decrease in the number of antifungal DDDs per 1000 hospitalization days (from 1100 DDD/PD in 2003 to 600 DDD/PD in 2011) in the haematology unit, with a smaller reduction elsewhere (400 to 300 DDD/PD). Stable frequency of IFIs
Mondain et al. (2013) [29]	1800-bed tertiary care hospital, Nice, France	ID, microbiology, pharmacy, and haemato-oncology specialists	Post-prescription review by AFS team with non-compulsory recommendations communicated to the physician in charge. Patients identified by prescription of high-cost antifungals (echinocandins, lipid formulations of amphotericin B, posaconazole, and voriconazole) or significant microbiological result. Onsite TDM and *Aspergillus* PCR introduced	Treatment and prophylaxis guidelines. Pharmacist prompt for IV to oral switch for fluconazole. On-site diagnostics (GM antigen, CT, bronchoscopy). Regular education and training. Order forms for echinocandins, voriconazole, posaconazole, lipid-based amphotericin	Improving diagnosis and de-escalation of therapy by advising all necessary mycological investigations	Recommendations made in 54% of reviews regarding: ♦ diagnosis (33%) ♦ serological investigations (41%) ♦ performing a CT scan (18%) ♦ TDM (30%) ♦ start therapy (4%) ♦ stop therapy (15%) ♦ switch therapy (30%) Advice acceptance 88% AF consumption and cost remained stable

ID, infectious diseases; AF, antifungal; IV, intravenous; DDD, defined daily dose; CVC, central venous catheter; LOS, length of stay; IFI, invasive fungal infection; TDM, therapeutic drug monitoring; PCR, polymerase chain reaction; GM, galactomannan; CT, computed tomography.

Source: data from Alfandari S et al. 2014 [26]; Apisarnthanarak A et al. 2010 [27]; López-Medrano F et al. 2013 [28]; Mondain V et al. 2013 [29]; Reed EE et al. 2014 [30].

Given the scarcity of supporting literature, AFS programmes should be implemented hand-in-hand with a strategy to demonstrate their performance. Parameters that should be prospectively monitored include: interventions made by the stewardship team and their acceptance rates, patient outcomes, drug consumption and expenditure, as well as additional costs of AFS such as staff time and implementation of additional diagnostic tests.

References

1 Ananda-Rajah MR, Slavin MA, Thursky KT. The case for antifungal stewardship. *Curr Opin Infect Dis* 2012;**25**:1–9.

2 Cleveland AA, Harrison LH, Farley MM, Hollick R, Stein B, Chiller TM, et al. Declining incidence of candidemia and the shifting epidemiology of *Candida* resistance in two US metropolitan areas, 2008–2013: results from population-based surveillance. *PLoS One* 2015;**10**:e0120452.

3 Denning DW, Park S, Lass-Florl C, Fraczek MG, Kirwan M, Gore R, et al. High-frequency triazole resistance found in nonculturable *Aspergillus fumigatus* from lungs of patients with chronic fungal disease. *Clin Infect Dis* 2011;**52**:1123–9.

4 Howard SJ, Cerar D, Anderson MJ, Albarrag A, Fisher MC, Pasqualotto AC, et al. Frequency and evolution of azole resistance in *Aspergillus fumigatus* associated with treatment failure. *Emerg Infect Dis* 2009;**15**:1068–76.

5 Wang E, Farmakiotis D, Yang D, McCue DA, Kantarjian HM, Kontoyiannis DP, et al. The ever-evolving landscape of candidaemia in patients with acute leukaemia: non-susceptibility to caspofungin and multidrug resistance are associated with increased mortality. *J Antimicrob Chemother* 2015;**70**:2362–8.

6 Kanamaru A, Tatsumi Y. Microbiological data for patients with febrile neutropenia. *Clin Infect Dis* 2004;**39**(S1):S7–S10.

7 MasiaCanuto M, Gutierrez Rodero F. Antifungal drug resistance to azoles and polyenes. *Lancet Infect Dis* 2002;**2**:550–63.

8 Pfaller MA, Diekema DJ, Gibbs DL, Newell VA, Meis JF, Gould IM, et al. Results from the ARTEMIS DISK Global Antifungal Surveillance study, 1997 to 2005: an 8.5-year analysis of susceptibilities of *Candida* species and other yeast species to fluconazole and voriconazole determined by CLSI standardized disk diffusion testing. *J Clin Microbiol* 2007;**45**:1735–45.

9 Valerio M, Munoz P, Zamora E, Salcedo M, Verde E, Bustinza A, et al. Stewardship in antifungals. How much do prescribing physicians know? Oral presentation at the 21st ECCMID/27th ICC. *ClinMicrob Infect* 2011;**17**(Suppl. 4):S35.

10 Pagano L, Caira M, Candoni A, Offidani M, Martino B, Specchia G, et al. Invasive aspergillosis in patients with acute myeloid leukemia: a SEIFEM-2008 registry study. *Haematologica* 2010;**95**:644–50.

11 Perkhofer S, Lass-Florl C, Hell M, Russ G, Krause R, Hönigl M, et al. The Nationwide Austrian Aspergillus Registry: a prospective data collection on epidemiology, therapy and outcome of invasive mould infections in immunocompromised and/or immunosuppressed patients. *Int J Antimicrob Agents* 2010;**36**:531–6.

12 Kontoyiannis DP, Marr KA, Park BJ, Alexander BD, Anaissie EJ, Walsh TJ, et al. Prospective surveillance for invasive fungal infections in hematopoietic stem cell transplant recipients, 2001–2006: overview of the Transplant-Associated Infection Surveillance Network (TRANSNET) Database. *Clin Infect Dis* 2010;**50**:1091–100.

13 Morrell M, Fraser VJ, Kollef MH. Delaying the empiric treatment of *Candida* bloodstream infection until positive blood culture results are obtained: a potential risk factor for hospital mortality. *Antimicrob Agents Chemother* 2005;**49**:3640–5.

14 Valerio M, Rodriguez-Gonzalez CG, Munoz P, Caliz B, Sanjurjo M, Bouza E, et al. Evaluation of antifungal use in a tertiary care institution: antifungal stewardship urgently needed. *J Antimicrob Chemother* 2014;**69**:1993–9.

15 **Shah DN, Yau R, Weston J, Lasco TM, Salazar M, Palmer HR, et al.** Evaluation of antifungal therapy in patients with candidaemia based on susceptibility testing results: implications for antimicrobial stewardship programmes. *J Antimicrob Chemother* 2011;**66**:2146–51.

16 **Aguado JM, Vázquez L, Fernández-Ruiz M, Villaescusa T, Ruiz-Camps I, Barba P, et al.** Serum galactomannan versus a combination of galactomannan and polymerase chain reaction-based *Aspergillus* DNA detection for early therapy of invasive aspergillosis in high-risk hematological patients: a randomized controlled trial. *Clin Infect Dis* 2015;**60**:405–14.

17 **Barnes RA, White PL, Bygrave C, Evans N, Healy B, Kell J.** Clinical impact of enhanced diagnosis of invasive fungal disease in high-risk haematology and stem cell transplant patients. *J Clin Pathol* 2009;**62**:64–9.

18 **Cordonnier C, Pautas C, Maury S, Vekhoff A, Farhat H, Suarez F, et al.** Empirical versus preemptive anti- fungal therapy for high-risk, febrile, neutropenic patients: a randomized, controlled trial. *Clin Infect Dis* 2009;**48**:1042–51.

19 **Maertens J, Theunissen K, Verhoef G, Verschakelen J, Lagrou K, Verbeken E, et al.** Galactomannan and computed tomography-based preemptive antifungal therapy in neutropenic patients at high risk for invasive fungal infection: a prospective feasibility study. *Clin Infect Dis* 2005;**41**:1242–50.

20 **Morrissey CO, Chen SCA, Sorrell TC, Milliken S, Bardy PG, Bradstock KF, et al.** Galactomannan and PCR versus culture and histology for directing use of antifungal treatment for invasive aspergillosis in high-risk haematology patients: a randomised controlled trial. *Lancet Infect Dis* 2013;**13**:519–28.

21 **Avni T, Leibovici L, Paul M.** PCR diagnosis of invasive candidiasis: systematic review and meta-analysis. *J Clin Microbiol* 2011;**49**:665–70.

22 **Dhiman N, Hall L, Wohlfiel SL, Buckwalter SP, Wengenack NL.** Performance and cost analysis of matrix-assisted laser desorption ionization-time of flight mass spectrometry for routine identification of yeast. *J Clin Microbiol* 2011;**49**:1614–16.

23 **Nguyen MH, Wissel MC, Shields RK, Salomoni MA, Hao B, Press EG, et al.** Performance of *Candida* real-time polymerase chain reaction, beta-d-glucan assay, and blood cultures in the diagnosis of invasive candidiasis. *Clin Infect Dis* 2012;**54**:1240–8.

24 **Marom EM, Kontoyiannis DP.** Imaging studies for diagnosing invasive fungal pneumonia in immunocompromised patients. *Curr Opin Infect Dis* 2011;**24**:309–14.

25 **Hardak E, Yigla M, Avivi I, Fruchter O, Sprecher H, Oren I.** Impact of PCR-based diagnosis of invasive pulmonary aspergillosis on clinical outcome. *Bone Marrow Transplant* 2009;**44**:595–9.

26 **Alfandari S, Berthon C, Coiteux V.** Antifungal stewardship: implementation in a French teaching hospital. *Med Mal Infect* 2014;**44**:154–8.

27 **Apisarnthanarak A, Yatrasert A, Mundy L.** Thammasat University Antimicrobial Stewardship Team. Impact of education and an antifungal stewardship program for candidiasis at a Thai tertiary care center. *Infect Control Hosp Epidemiol* 2010;**31**:722–7.

28 **López-Medrano F, San Juan R, Lizasoain M, Catalán M, Ferrari JM, Chaves F, et al.** A non-compulsory stewardship programme for the management of antifungals in a university-affiliated hospital. *Clin Microbiol Infect* 2013;**19**:56–61.

29 **Mondain V, Lieutier F, Hasseine L, Gari-Toussaint M, Poiree M, Lions C, et al.** A 6-year antifungal stewardship programme in a teaching hospital. *Infection* 2013;**41**:621–8.

30 **Reed EE, West JE, Keating EA, Pancholi P, Balada-Llasat J-M, Mangino JE, et al.** Improving the management of candidemia through antimicrobial stewardship interventions. *Diagn Microbiol Infect Dis* 2014;**78**:157–61.

31 **Whitney L, Al-Ghusein H, Koh M, Klammer M, Bicanic T.** Antifungal stewardship at a London teaching hospital achieves sustained cost reduction over 3 years without compromising microbiologic and clinical outcomes. Oral presentation at the 24th ECCMID 2014. Abstract available from: http://2014.eccmid.org/

32 **Parkinson C, Gilchrist M, Armstrong-Jones D, Whitney L, Bicanic T.** Sharing and developing a consensus approach to anti-fungal stewardship in London—a proof of concept. Poster presentation at the Federation of Infection Societies Annual Conference, 2014, Harrogate.

Chapter 17

Near-patient testing, infection biomarkers, and rapid diagnostics

Matthew Dryden

Introduction to near-patient testing, infection biomarkers, and rapid diagnostics

Antibiotic prescribing runs along a therapeutic knife-edge: withholding antibiotics could lead to worsening infection or death, while over-prescribing leads to resistance. There is huge variation in prescribing habits between nations, institutions, units, practices, and individual prescribers, and this variance can rarely be attributed to differences in the incidence of infection or clinical presentation. It is rather associated with differences in culture, diagnostic facilities, medical training, economic factors, and attitudes to risk. Over-prescribing of antimicrobials is the selection pressure that leads to antibiotic resistance, and if this is combined with poor community public health and inadequate infection prevention in healthcare facilities, then resistant microbes proliferate as colonizers and then become pathogens. Resistance is now a global health hazard which, like a runaway juggernaut, is going to prove near impossible to control.

Microbiological diagnostics today would still seem very familiar to their nineteenth-century discoverers. A sample of infected tissue is collected and grown on agar plates and growth, if it occurs, takes a day or two or more. Then antibiotic sensitivity testing has to be carried out, which means that a meaningful result to guide antibiotic treatment may take from 1 day at best to more than 5 days. Treating a patient cannot wait for the result, and so where antibiotic prescribing is well controlled, carefully designed antibiotic guidelines offer the most appropriate empiric antibiotic therapy. Where antibiotic prescribing is poorly controlled, anything goes. A solution to the whole issue would be to have rapid diagnostic tests, which in a short period of time could confirm the diagnosis and support prescribing or withholding antibiotics. Some such tests already exist.

An example of effective rapid diagnostics assisting antibiotic use is *Chlamydia trachomatis* infection. Infection of the genital tract with *C. trachomatis* is common and often asymptomatic. A public health programme could decide to treat all those at risk in case they had the infection. This would lead to overuse of antibiotics. Instead, those at risk can take a urine sample to a diagnostic centre where a rapid polymerase chain reaction (PCR) test for *C. trachomatis* DNA is performed. If this test is positive the patient is treated with an antibiotic; if negative, antibiotic is withheld. This process is clear, simple, and without ambiguity. Medicine is rarely so straightforward, and in more complex clinical scenarios it is likely that rapid diagnosis will involve an algorithm of clinical signs and predictive diagnostic tests.

What should rapid diagnostic tests detect?

Identification of the presence of bacterial infection

Establishing the presence of bacterial infection would be clinically useful to ensure that the patient receives appropriate antibiotics early, and it is important from the viewpoint of antimicrobial stewardship that patients without bacterial infection do not receive antibiotics. Biomarkers are helpful here. Rapid detection of a neutrophilia or raised C-reactive protein (CRP) has long been used to aid a diagnosis of infection and support antibiotic use. Procalcitonin (PCT) appears to be a more sensitive marker of bacterial infection. In a study which included medical and critical care patients with possible but doubtful infection, antibiotics were withheld if the bedside PCT was below the cut-off value. Patients who had antibiotics withheld did not develop infection or require antibiotics. Empiric antibiotic use was reduced by a half in this group [1]. In a randomized open-label trial in an intensive care unit (ICU) the use of the PCT marker for starting and stopping antibiotics significantly reduced antibiotic consumption without any change in mortality [2]. A meta-analysis of randomized clinical trials involving ICU patients with different diagnoses showed that the use of PCT levels appears to safely and significantly decrease antimicrobial use in the ICU and may also decrease the length of stay in the ICU [3]. A table of PCT values to guide starting and continuation of antibiotics is now widely used (see Table 17.1).

A novel technology called enzymatic template generation and amplification (ETGA) has been developed to detect live bacteria and fungi in normally sterile clinical specimens, such as blood. The technology has been shown to detect microorganisms by the activity of microbial enzymes (specifically, DNA polymerases) which can be measured by real-time PCR (qPCR) in a simple detection reaction that produces a measurable fluorescent signal. This technology has been assessed in a clinical environment and shown to give a high negative predictive value for a negative blood culture within hours of collection, theoretically allowing discontinuation of antibiotics [4].

Table 17.1 Guidelines for antibiotic management based on PCT (if collected early in illness, repeat test at 6–12 hours). Severe unequivocal sepsis is excluded

(a) Starting antibiotics

PCT concentration			
<0.25 µg/L	0.25–0.5	0.5–1.0 µg/L	>1.0 µg/L
Antibiotic strongly discouraged	Antibiotic discouraged	Antibiotic encouraged	Antibiotic strongly encouraged

(b) Stopping antibiotics

PCT concentration			
<0.25 µg/L	PCT decrease by >80% from peak OR 0.25–0.5 µg/L	PCT decrease by <80% from peak AND >0.5 µg/L	PCT increase from peak AND >0.5 µg/L
Stopping antibiotic strongly encouraged	Stopping antibiotic encouraged	Continue antibiotic	Review diagnosis and consider changing antibiotic

Other technology is proving useful during surgical procedures. Detection of α-defensin in joint fluid in native joints and in revision surgery can aid management decisions concerning antibiotic use and surgical requirements [5].

Most antibiotics are used in primary care. The use of biomarkers during the consultation to reduce antibiotic prescribing would have a major effect on consumption. CRP testing has been used in primary care to predict requirement for antibiotics, and this has been most successful in predicting requirement for antibiotics in respiratory infection [6]. In primary care, there are challenges in fitting delivery of a near-patient test into a short consultation. New technologies delivering near-patient testing of other biomarkers (PCT and pro-adrenomedullin) require assessment in primary care.

The cause of the infection

There are a few effective tests that can diagnose at the bedside the identity of bacteria causing infection that can also support antimicrobial stewardship. Rapid antigen tests for *Streptococcus* Group A or PCR for meticillin-resistant *Staphylococcus aureus* (MRSA) colonization can influence antibiotic use but do not definitively identify the cause of infection. Rapid urinary antigen detection for pneumococcus or *Legionella pneumophila* can achieve rapid diagnosis. Malaria antigen detection can be applied directly to a blood sample. Rapid PCR for *Clostridium difficile* infection or norovirus can assist timely management of infection control precautions and antibiotic management in hospitals.

Most other tests for early identification of the pathogen and early sensitivity testing require preliminary culture growth or a positive blood culture. There are several molecular techniques for the identification of specific pathogens once the sample (usually blood culture) signals positive growth [7]. It has been estimated that the average time for a microbiology laboratory to deliver the result of an organism identification and susceptibility test is 40 hours. These techniques include PCR, multiplex PCR, nanoparticle probe technology (nucleic acid extraction and PCR amplification), and peptide nucleic acid fluorescent *in situ* hybridization (PNA FISH). They allow rapid identification of certain specific pathogens and some resistance genes, for example *mecA*, within minutes to hours of culture positivity. However, the range of organisms identified depends on the test and is not universal. Matrix-assisted laser desorption/ionization time-of-flight mass spectrometry (MALDI-TOF) is an automated system that allows rapid identification of most organisms from culture. The generated mass spectrum provides a profile or fingerprint of the organism that is compared with those of well-characterized organisms in a database. These rapid results can support an antimicrobial stewardship programme and aid early rationalization of prescribing.

Resolution

Biomarkers can identify when the patient has responded to treatment and no longer requires antibiotics. Serial PCT measurement has been used to establish the earliest point at which antimicrobials can be safely discontinued [8]. A reduction in antibiotic duration could aid antimicrobial stewardship by reducing selection pressure on bacteria and possibly reduce rates of resistance. Antibiotic duration has been reduced without the requirement for biomarkers, but they remain useful in individual cases.

Prognosis

PCT has been used to predict prognosis. In a number of large studies in intensive care, a high maximum PCT and an increase in PCT value following the first reading >1.0 ng/mL were both independent predictors of 90-day mortality [8]. The relative risk for mortality increased with

---

Box 17.1 Technology available for achieving rapid diagnostics

1. Molecular diagnosis to identify the pathogen *in situ* or once cultured: MALDI-TOF, PCR, multiplex PCR, nanoparticle probe technology, PNA FISH, automated optical systems such as VITEK

2. Molecular diagnosis to determine antimicrobial susceptibility: PCR, multiplex PCR, nanoparticle probe technology, automated real-time PCR, VITEK

3. Molecular diagnosis to determine the presence of bacterial infection: Momentum Cognitor ETGA

4. Molecular diagnosis to determine the absence of bacterial infection: Momentum Cognitor ETGA

5. Biomarkers to predict the presence of bacterial infection: PCT, CRP, pro-adrenomedullin, α-defensin

6. Biomarkers to predict the course of the infection: CRP, PCT, pro-adrenomedullin

7. Metabolomics to predict the presence of infection: this is in its infancy for the detection of infection as opposed to the identification of cultured bacteria

Source: data from *Hampshire Hospitals NHS Foundation Trust Antibiotic Guidelines 2014*, Copyright © Department of Microbiology for Basingstoke and North Hampshire Foundation Trust Hospital 2014.

---

every day for which the PCT value continued to rise after the first reading >1.0 ng/mL. The clinical use of biomarkers as a prognostic indicator is unclear as they are unlikely to affect day to day patient management or antibiotic management (Box 17.1).

Limitations

Rapid diagnostics are only useful if they are acted upon in a timely manner and are used to educate staff caring for the patient. They can rarely replace clinical judgement. Their use must be incorporated into a clear patient management plan. They should also be used in conjunction with careful clinical assessment and incorporated into management algorithms. Some tests can be too sensitive and identify the presence of pathogens that need not necessarily be causing disease.

Rapid diagnostic methods have huge potential as a multidisciplinary tool bringing together the clinician, diagnostician, pharmacist, hospital manager, and infection prevention personnel in the improved management of the patient in primary and secondary care. Although at present there is no substitute for clinical judgement, diagnostic technology is advancing at a rapid pace, and for the optimist diagnostic tools are the best hope for ensuring the optimal use of antibiotics in the

---

Box 17.2 Practical points

Molecular diagnostics and biomarkers can support antimicrobial stewardship:

+ in the requirement for antibiotics
+ in starting antibiotics
+ in the duration of antibiotics
+ in stopping antibiotics
+ in assessing prognosis

future. Rapid diagnostics, including molecular methods and biomarkers, can play a real role in supporting antimicrobial stewardship by supporting clinical judgement on the requirement for, the commencement of, and the duration of treatment and the cessation of antibiotics (Box 17.2).

References

1 **Saeed K, Dryden MS, Bourne S, Paget C, Proud A.** Reduction in antibiotic use through procalcitonin testing in patients in the medical admission unit or intensive care unit with suspicion of infection. *J Hosp Infect* 2011;78:289–92.

2 **Bouadma L, Luyt CE, Tubach F, Cracco C, Alvarez A, Schwebel C, et al.** Use of procalcitonin to reduce patients' exposure to antibiotics in intensive care units (PRORATA trial): a multicentre randomised controlled trial. *Lancet* 2010;375:463–74.

3 **Agarwal R, Schwartz DN.** Procalcitonin to guide duration of antimicrobial therapy in intensive care units: a systematic review. *Clin Infect Dis* 2011;53:379–87.

4 **Crow M, Bennett HV, Grover M, Dryden MS.** Evaluation of a new method for the rapid exclusion of infection in suspected bacteraemia. Poster presentation at the 24th ECCMID 2014. Poster and abstract available from: http://2014.eccmid.org/

5 **Deirmengian C, Kardos K, Kilmartin P, Cameron A, Schiller K, Parvizi J.** Combined measurement of synovial fluid α-defensin and CRP level. *J Bone Joint Surg Am* 2014;96:1439–45.

6 **Cals JW, Schot MJ, de Jong SA, Dinant GJ, Hopstaken RM.** Point-of-care C-reactive protein testing and antibiotic prescribing for respiratory tract infections: a randomized controlled trial. *Ann Fam Med* 2010;8:124–33.

7 **Bauer K, Perez K, Forrest G, Goff DA.** Review of rapid diagnostic tests used by antimicrobial stewardship programs. *Clin Infect Dis* 2014;59(Suppl. 3):S134–S145.

8 **Kibe S, Adams K, Barlow G.** Diagnostic and prognostic biomarkers of sepsis in critical care. *J Antimicrob Chemother* 2011;66(Suppl. 2):ii33–ii40.

Chapter 18

Antimicrobial stewardship in a resource-poor setting

Marc Mendelson

Introduction to antimicrobial stewardship in a resource-poor setting

Antimicrobial resistance hits low- and middle-income countries (LMICs) hardest—of the projected 10 million deaths per year from antimicrobial-resistant infections that will occur by 2050 the hammer blow will fall hardest on resource-poor LMICs in Asia and Africa (Figure 18.1). The reason for this geographical variation is multifactorial, but the main influence is the significant burden of infection in LMICs, necessitating high levels of antimicrobial use. Indeed, in the last 10 years, 75% of the 36% global increase in human antibiotic consumption has been driven by just five LMICs, Brazil, Russia, India, China, and South Africa (the BRICS nations) [1]. An inability to directly address the social determinants of disease predisposes populations in LMICs to infection; poor water and sanitation (diarrhoeal diseases), overcrowding [respiratory infections, such as pneumonia and tuberculosis (TB)], close co-habitation with animals (zoonoses), and weakened immune systems through high levels of malnutrition due to poverty or to human immunodeficiency virus (HIV) infection.

Coupled to the challenge of a high burden of infection is the lack of access to infection prevention instruments such as vaccination and even simpler, cheap interventions such as soap for hand washing that could negate the need for antimicrobials in the first place.

Successful stewardship requires access to affordable, assured-quality antimicrobials and the tools required to enable appropriate use

Currently, more children under the age of 5 years in LMICs die from pneumonia due to lack of access to antibiotic treatment than due to antibiotic resistance [2]. Furthermore, access to antibiotics depends on wealth; more children in the top quintiles of households (based on wealth) will receive antibiotics than those in the bottom quintiles [3]. A range of novel financing initiatives has been developed to try to increase access to affordable vaccines and antimicrobials in LMICs at country level, mainly targeting HIV, tuberculosis, and malaria [4]. Such funding mechanisms could be adapted to increase access for other antimicrobials, including antibiotics. LMICs with weak health systems and poorly regulated medicines control bodies often fall prey to substandard and falsified antimicrobials, which drive resistance through sub-optimal action [5].

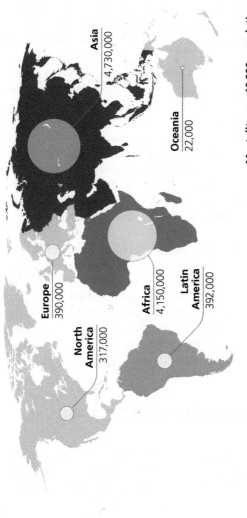

Figure 18.1 Deaths attributable to antimicrobial resistance per year by 2050.

Major global initiatives to ensure appropriate prescribing for specific infections have reduced the risk of resistance, but they remain examples of vertical 'siloed' initiatives. The Global Fund-led Affordable Medicines Facility—Malaria successfully negotiated price reductions for artemisinin combination therapies [6] with the aim of reducing the use of artemisinin monotherapy, one driver of increasing artemisinin resistance in Southeast Asia. In 2014, a $60 million grant from UNITAID ensured accelerated uptake of two new antimycobacterials, bedaquiline and delamanid, in 17 countries, expanding access to newer, more effective treatments for multidrug-resistant (MDR) TB [7]. The Green Light Committee initiative, a partnership founded in 2006 by the World Health Organization and the Stop TB Partnership and subsequently developed into a global framework, has provided financial and technical assistance to LMICs to support expansion of MDR TB services and care [8]. Lessons from such initiatives could be equally applicable to antibiotic access programmes.

Diagnostic uncertainty is a key driver of antibiotic overuse. Access to diagnostic tests, preferably rapid and point of care (POC) that can optimize antimicrobial management, is an essential stewardship tool for LMICs; the availability of a rapid diagnostic test for malaria led to a four-fold reduction in antimalarial use and a five-fold increase in appropriate antibiotic use [9]. A new POC urine liporarabinomanan strip test is particularly useful in the diagnosis of TB in HIV–TB co-infected patients with advanced immunosuppression [10]. When bacterial identification and information on resistance is combined, delay to appropriate antimicrobial use may be reduced. Xpert MTB/RIF (Cepheid, Sunnyvale, CA, USA), an automated, real-time nucleic acid amplification system, detects rifampicin-resistant pulmonary [11] and extrapulmonary TB [12] within 2 hours. However, the rollout of such technology in many LMICs and its high cost remains a considerable challenge [13].

Weak health systems, limited human resources, and poor infrastructure in LMICs have necessitated novel community models of care that simplify management of infection and make prescribing uniform. Integrated community case management (iCCM), an equity-focused strategy to improve access for children to essential services, has been highly successful at shifting prescribing from doctors to community health workers [14] and in increasing the appropriateness of antimicrobial prescribing [15–17]. Similarly, integrated management of childhood illness (IMCI) and its adult counterpart, integrated management of adolescent and adult illness (IMAI), have empowered and trained healthcare workers (HCWs) and influenced appropriate prescribing [18].

Which antimicrobial stewardship interventions work in LMICs?

Two Cochrane database reviews detail the result of antimicrobial stewardship (AMS) interventions at community [19] and hospital [20] level. Of the 39 outpatient interventions reported, only six were conducted in LMICs [19], with similarly low numbers represented in the hospital studies, none of which were conducted in Africa [20]. Hence, there are few data to guide us with regard to what works in LMICs, and much is extrapolated from studies in high-income settings. Generally, restrictive interventions such as removal of antimicrobials, compulsory prescription forms, expert approval, or specialist review and making change are more successful at reducing antimicrobial prescribing in the short term (the first 6 months), but are no better than persuasive interventions (educational materials and outreach, reminders, or audit and feedback) in the long term (12–24 months).

Non-prescription use of antimicrobials is associated with very short courses and inappropriate drug choice, and accounts for 19–100% of antimicrobial use in LMICs [21]. However, pharmacists

> **Box 18.1 Restricting over-the-counter antibiotic sales in India—the Chennai Declaration**
>
> The Chennai Declaration was adopted following a joint meeting of the medical societies of India in 2012. It came as a response to a non-implementable national antibiotic policy 1 year previously that had called for all antibiotics to require a prescription. The Chennai Declaration covers a wide range of interventions to be implemented, yet control of OTC prescribing of antibiotics has been a major initial focus. Until publication and implementation of the declaration, there was no restriction on OTC dispensing without prescription [24]. The declaration stated that India needs 'an implementable antibiotic policy' and not 'a perfect policy' [22]. With this in mind, the 5-year timeline for implementation of India's OTC policy has included 24 high-end antibiotics and antimycobacterials used for the treatment of TB for addition to the restricted list of medicines within the first year. A registry of these antibiotic sales is to be kept for 3 years. The 2-year and 5-year targets are 60% and 90% of antibiotics to be included in the restricted list, respectively [23].
>
> Source: data from Ghafur A et al. 2012 [22]; Chennai Declaration Team 2014 [23]; and Rathnakar UP et al. 2012 [24].

may be the major provider of antimicrobials where prescribers are scarce, such as rural areas. A recent effort to restrict non-prescription over-the-counter (OTC) antibiotic sales has been undertaken in India as part of the Chennai Declaration (Box 18.1) [22,23].

This effort is not without many challenges, but in a country such as India, where all forms of antibiotics were available OTC, including 'high-end' injectable antibiotics, this ambitious project forms the first of a set of key stewardship interventions.

What does a successful antimicrobial resistance programme look like in LMICs?

India is joined by a number of LMICs that have started to put national antimicrobial resistance plans in place. Many common themes are recognized, particularly the standard approaches of improving surveillance and reporting, AMS, and infection prevention that form the bedrock of national interventions (Figure 18.2).

A national situational analysis as a first step to identify individual country challenges is of critical importance. In this regard the Global Antibiotic Resistance Partnership (GARP) has been a vital catalyst to many LMIC programmes; both the South African National Strategy Framework on AMR [25] and the Viet Nam Resistance Project (VINARES) [26] began with GARP-led situational analyses in the human and animal sectors. VINARES (Box 18.2) stands as an excellent example of how good multilevel governance can have a positive impact on a national AMR strategy.

Lessons from South Africa

As part of a situational analysis, it is important to understand the barriers that exist, including society-specific behaviours and competing health challenges, which may need to be addressed before an AMS programme can be implemented; HIV overwhelmed the South African health landscape for decades, and it was not until a comprehensive antiretroviral treatment programme was under way that the focus could move on to other threats.

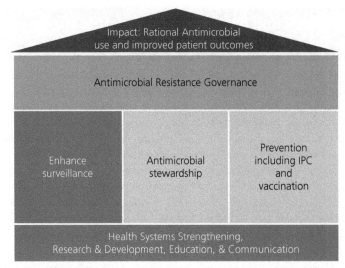

Figure 18.2 The pillars of a national antimicrobial resistance programme (IPC, infection prevention and control).

Reproduced courtesy of the South Africa National Department of Health.

Successful AMR programmes rely on a multidisciplinary, coordinated group to champion change, a particular challenge for LMICs that lack infectious diseases specialists and microbiologists. However, such is the burden of infection in most LMICs that non-specialists are often equipped to play this role. The South African Antibiotic Stewardship Programme (SAASP) was formed to champion and drive change at the coalface and to partner the National Department of Health. SAASP was strategically positioned under the auspices of the Federation of Infectious Diseases Societies of Southern Africa, the national umbrella organization for infection societies, to access key role-players in adult and paediatric infectious diseases, clinical microbiology, infection prevention and control, travel medicine, and sexually transmitted diseases. A multidisciplinary working group provides governance. Partnership with the South

---

Box 18.2 The Viet Nam Resistance (VINARES) Project

Despite adequate legislation to tackle AMR in Viet Nam, a lack of resources to implement effective policy enforcement was identified, and led to the VINARES project, a public–private partnership including international collaborators, to implement AMR containment strategies. Sixteen hospitals participated to address infection control, healthcare-associated infections, antibiotic consumption, and microbiological surveillance and reporting. Information and quality control systems were added to support the work, including simple pharmacy databases to define monthly antibiotic consumption and surveillance database software for the microbiology laboratories. The strength of the project is underpinned by its research focus in identifying areas for improvement before consultation and implementation, with a strong training component, and by its focus on capacity development to equip hospitals to deliver self-sufficient antimicrobial stewardship long-term.

Source: data from Chennai Declaration Team, 'Chennai Declaration: 5-year plan to tackle the challenge of anti-microbial resistance', *Indian Journal of Medical Microbiology*, Volume 32, Issue 3, pp. 221–8, Copyright © 2014.

African Society of Clinical Pharmacy recognizes the pivotal role of pharmacists, a cadre of HCWs able to form the nucleus of a stewardship team. Other skill sets represented in SAASP include critical care specialists, surgeons, quality improvement specialists, and epidemiologists. South Africa is fortunate to have a strong group of veterinary infection experts, who complete the team.

Advocacy and engagement with national government were early objectives, and having briefed the minister of health, immediate action followed to develop a national working group, led by the director general of health. Leadership from the highest level is a vital component of any change programme, and South Africa's success is a direct result of such leadership; all stakeholders signed the national AMR strategy framework commitments in 2014 (Figure 18.3). These have been reinforced by national core standards for AMS and infection prevention overseen by the Office of Health Standards Compliance. Each hospital will be required to have an antibiotic stewardship committee and team(s).

The importance of international collaboration for resource-poor countries is a valuable lesson. The surveillance and reporting structures of both Viet Nam and South Africa have benefitted from international collaboration on data processing and integration, and are set to benefit further from AMR work streams within the Global Health Security Agenda [27].

For South Africa, collaboration with the Center for Disease Dynamics and Economic Policy has led to the production of an AMR map, which will help inform appropriate empiric national prescribing choice.

Stewardship programmes are now widespread across public and private institutions in many provinces, concentrating on 'low-hanging fruit' interventions [28]. The success of such programmes in individual institutions is an important motivator for change elsewhere, and the importance of feedback at national conferences and the publication of results cannot be overstated. The development of specific tools to facilitate appropriate prescribing is a useful intervention; in South Africa, an open access antibiotic prescription chart, which also enables audit and research, has been developed [29]. Rolling out stewardship to under-resourced provinces is a challenge and one that is being addressed by developing national centres for AMS to 'train the trainer'. Furthermore work is ongoing with the Health Professions Council of South Africa towards an antibiotic prescribing 'licence' that will involve a web-based course and examination that all prescribers must undergo and be re-validated biennially.

Infection prevention, re-aligning the curriculum of school learners, medical, and paramedical students, continuing professional development for doctors, nurses, and ancillary HCW, and finally development of public awareness campaigns need to be country-specific and take into account social and behavioural norms, but their messages and content are not unique to South Africa.

Antimicrobial stewardship in resource-poor settings: where next?

AMS programmes in LMICs need to be context specific and their format will be influenced by many factors, including level of expertise, human resources, infrastructure, and competing health and economic interests. Performance of a situational analysis allows identification of important areas of focus and where opportunities for collaboration to strengthen efforts may be needed. Measurement is vital to appraise interventions and to indicate where further resources are required. The WHO Global Action Plan [30] provides guidance on the essential components of a national strategy, and is a useful starting point for any LMIC.

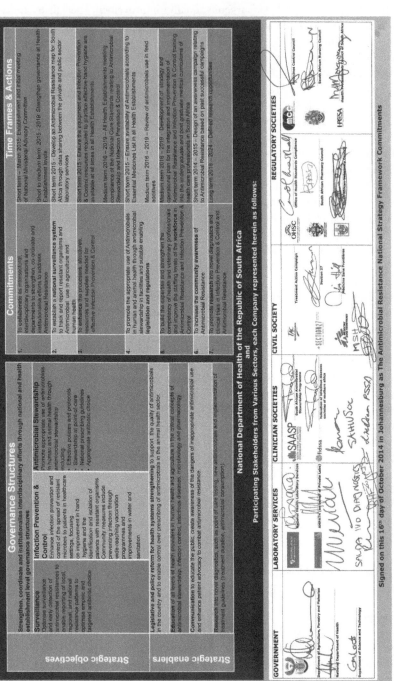

Figure 18.3 South Africa's National Strategy Framework Commitments.

Reproduced courtesy of the South Africa National Department of Health.

References

1 Van Boeckel TP, Gandra S, Ashok A, Caudron Q, Grenfell BT, Levin SA, et al. Global antibiotic consumption 2000 to 2010: an analysis of national pharmaceutical sales data. *Lancet Infect Dis* 2014;**14**:742–50.

2 Laxminarayan R, Duse A, Wattal C, Zaidi AK, Wertheim HF, Sumpradit N, et al. Antibiotic resistance-the need for global solutions. *Lancet Infect Dis* 2013;**13**:1057–98. [Errata in *Lancet Infect Dis* 2014;**14**:182 and 2014;14:11.]

3 Johansson EW, Carvajal L, Newby H, Young M, Wardlaw T. *Pneumonia and diarrhoea: tackling the deadliest diseases for the world's poorest children*. 2012. New York: UNICEF.

4 Atun R, Knaul FM, Akachi Y, Frenk J. Innovative financing for health: what is truly innovative? *Lancet* 2012;**380**:2044–9.

5 Kelesidis T, Falagas ME. Substandard/counterfeit antimicrobial drugs. *Clin Microbiol Rev* 2015;**28**:443–64.

6 Tougher S, Ye Y, Amuasi JH, Kourgueni IA, Thomson R, Goodman C, et al. Effect of the Affordable Medicines Facility—malaria (AMFm) on the availability, price, and market share of quality-assured artemisinin-based combination therapies in seven countries: a before-and-after analysis of outlet survey data. *Lancet* 2012;**380**:1916–26.

7 UNITAID. UNITAID approves grants of $160 million [internet]. 6 May 2014. Available from: http://www.unitaid.org/en/resources/press-centre/releases/1352-unitaid-approves-grants-of-160-million·

8 Case Studies for Global Health. Public and private partnership helps to set the standard of care for multi-drug resistant tuberculosis. 30 October 2009. Available at: http://casestudiesforglobalhealth.org/post.cfm/public-and-private-partnership-helps-to-set-the-standard-of-care-for-multi-drug-resistant-tuberculosis-1 (updated May 2012, accessed 14 March 2015).

9 Yeboah-Antwi K, Pilangana P, MacLeod WB, Semrau K, Siazeele K, Kalesha P, et al. Community case management of fever due to malaria and pneumonia in children under five in Zambia: a cluster randomized controlled trial. *PLoS Med* 2010;**7**(9):e1000340.

10 Peter JG, Theron G, Dheda K. Can point-of-care urine LAM strip testing for tuberculosis add value to clinical decision making in hospitalized HIV-infected persons? *PLoS ONE* 2013;**8**(2):e54875.

11 Boehme CC, Nabeta P, Hillemann D, Rapid molecular detection of tuberculosis and rifampin resistance. *New Engl J Med* 2010;**363**:1005–15.

12 Maynard-Smith L, Larke N, Peters JA, Lawn SD. Diagnostic accuracy of the Xpert MTB/RIF assay for extrapulmonary and pulmonary tuberculosis when testing non-respiratory samples: a systematic review. *BMC Infect Dis* 2014;**14**:709.

13 Denkinger C. Kik S, Pai M. Robust, reliable and resilient: designing molecular tuberculosis tests for microscopy centres in developing countries. *Expert Rev Mol Diag* 2013;**13**:763–7.

14 Callaghan M, Ford N, Schneider H. A systematic review of task-shifting for HIV treatment and care in Africa. *Hum Resour Health* 2010;**8**:8.

15 Gill CJ, Phiri-Mazala G, Guerina NG, Kasimba J, Mulenga M, MacLeod WB, et al. Effect of training traditional birth attendants on neonatal mortality (Lufwanyama Neonatal Survival Project): randomised controlled study. *Br Med J* 2011;**342**:d346.

16 Bang AT, Bang RA, Baitule SB, Reddy MH, Deshmukh MD. Effect of home-based neonatal care and management of sepsis on neonatal mortality: field trial in rural India. *Lancet* 1999;**354**:1955–61.

17 Hamer DH, Brooks ET, Semrau K, Pilangana P, MacLeod WB, Siazeele K, et al. Quality and safety of integrated community case management of malaria using rapid diagnostic tests and pneumonia by community health workers. *Pathog Glob Health* 2012;**106**:32–9.

18 Gouws E, Bryce J, Habicht J, Amaral J, Pariyo G, Schellenberg JA, et al. Improving antimicrobial use among health workers in first- level facilities : results from the Multi-Country Evaluation of the Integrated Management of Childhood Illness strategy. *Bull World Health Organ* 2004;**82**:509–15.

19 **Arnold SR, Straus SE.** Interventions to improve antibiotic prescribing practices in ambulatory care. *Cochrane Database Syst Rev* 2005;(4):CD003539.

20 **Davey P, Brown E, Charani E, Fenelon L, Gould IM, Holmes A, et al.** Interventions to improve antibiotic prescribing practices for hospital inpatients. *Cochrane Database Syst Rev* 2013;(4):CD003543.

21 **Morgan DJ, Okeke IN, Laxminarayan R, Perencevich EN, Weisenberg S.** Non-prescription antimicrobial use worldwide: a systematic review. *Lancet Infect Dis* 2011;**11**:692–701.

22 **Ghafur A, Mathai D, Muruganathan A, Jayalal JA, Kant R, Chaudhary D, et al.** The Chennai Declaration: a roadmap to tackle the challenge of antimicrobial resistance. *Indian J Cancer* 2012;**49**:84–94.

23 **Chennai Declaration Team.** 'Chennai Declaration': 5-year plan to tackle the challenge of anti-microbial resistance. *Indian J Med Microbiol* 2014;**32**:221–8.

24 **Rathnakar UP, Sharma NK, Garg R, Unnikrishnan B, Gopalakrishna HN.** A study on the sale of antimicrobial agents without prescriptions in pharmacies in an urban area in south India. *J Clin Diagn Res* 2012;**6**:951–4.

25 **Department of Health, Republic of South Africa.** Antimicrobial Resistance National Strategy Framework 2014–2024. Available at: http://www.health.gov.za (accessed 13 April 2015).

26 **Wertheim HF, Chandna A, Vu PD, Pham CV, Nguyen PD, Lam YM, et al.** Providing impetus, tools, and guidance to strengthen national capacity for antimicrobial stewardship in Viet Nam. *PLoS Med* 2013;**10**(5):e1001429.

27 **United States Department of Health and Human Services.** The Global Health Security Agenda. Available at: http://www.globalhealth.gov/global-health-topics/global-health-security/ghsagenda.html (accessed 13 April 2015).

28 **Boyles TH, Whitelaw A, Bamford C, Moodley M, Bonorchis K, Morris V, et al.** Antibiotic stewardship ward rounds and a dedicated prescription chart reduce antibiotic consumption and pharmacy costs without affecting inpatient mortality or re-admission rates. *PLoS ONE* 2013;**8**(12):e79747.

29 **South African Antibiotic Stewardship Programme.** Antibiotic Prescription Chart. Available at: http://www.fidssa.co.za/Content/Documents/SAASP_Antibiotic_Prescription_Chart_Oct_2014.pdf (accessed 3rd February 2016).

30 **World Health Organization.** *Antimicrobial resistance. Draft global action plan for antimicrobial resistance.* **2014.** Available at http://apps.who.int/gb/ebwha/pdf_files/EB136/B136_20-en.pdf (accessed 13 April 2015).

Index